Headaches

Carpal Tunnel Syndrome

Fibromyalgia

Dr. David M. Warwick

Doctor of Chiropractic

What Do These Symptoms Have In Common?

A very simple and straight forward answer to this complex question is that they all require a multi-faceted health care approach. There is not one single right answer or method when approaching these complex conditions. A team of health practitioners will offer you diverse methods and approaches that come from many different angles with each opinion complimenting the next. Each individual may experience one or all of these symptoms, and by utilizing many methods and practitioners (each offering their unique professional opinion and approaches based upon research, experience and methods), patients may find relief. All, some, or none of this information can be right for you, as you are an individual. Whether you have tried medicine, naturopathy, acupuncture, chiropractic, physical therapy, massage, yoga, exercise, or nutrition, there is one method that stands out in my mind after years of working with individuals suffering with headaches, carpal tunnel or fibromyalgia: a team-approach that YOU find moves you toward health and away from a dis-ease state. Not one blood study, saliva test, doctor's opinion, or feedback test will give you that ONE answer. I have seen individuals embrace multi-facet approaches and move along the wellness spectrum to a better quality of health and life. And while I see individuals having measurable changes with other methods or modalities, the one method most embraced and the primary approach for continued support for those suffering with these conditions was ... *Chiropractic*. As my patients will tell you, I do not believe there is one right path but when utilizing multiple methods of Chiropractic techniques, working with other health care providers on concurrent care, and having a close communicative approach with each individual, my patients receive measurable results that many times exceeds my expectations as well as theirs. I am happy to share the insights of this book and invite you to open yourself to the many healing possibilities there for you. Never give up hope – for your health now and into the future!

Yours In Health, Dr. David M. Warwick

Table of Contents

Headaches / Migraines

CARPAL TUNNEL SYNDROMES (CTS)

FIBROMYALGIA

HEADACHES / MIGRAINES

Can Chiropractic Help My Headaches?

According to the World Health Organization, headaches are among the most common disorders of the nervous system affecting an estimated 47% of adults during the past year. Headaches place a significant burden on both quality of life (personal, social, and occupational) and financial health. They are usually misdiagnosed by healthcare practitioners, and in general, are underestimated, under-recognized, and under-treated around the world. So, what about chiropractic and headaches... Does it help?

Suffice it to say, there are MANY studies showing chiropractic care helps headache sufferers. For instance, in a review of past research studies using an "evidence-based" approach, chiropractic treatment of adults with different types of headaches revealed very positive findings! Researchers note that chiropractic care helps those with episodic or chronic migraine headaches, cervicogenic headache (that is, headaches caused by neck problems), and tension-type headaches (chronic more than episodic). There appears to be additional benefit when chiropractic adjustments are combined with massage, mobilization, and/or adding certain types of exercises, although this was not consistently studied. In the studies that discussed adverse or negative effects of treatment, the researchers noted no serious adverse effects.

In patients suffering from athletic injuries, particularly post-concussion headache (PC-HA), chiropractic care can play a very important role in the patient's recovery. With an estimated 1.6 to 3.8 million sports-related brain injuries occurring each year, approximately 136,000 involve young high school athletes (although some argue this is "grossly underestimated").

11

Several published case studies report significant benefits for post-concussion patients after receiving chiropractic care, some of which included PC-HA from motor vehicle collisions, as well as from slips and falls. For example, one described an improvement in symptoms that included deficits in short-term memory as well as attention problems. In this particular study, a six-year-old boy fell from a slide in the playground, and after 18 months of continuous problems, underwent a course of chiropractic care. After just three weeks of care, his spelling test scores improved from 20% to 80% with even more benefits observed by the eighth week of care!

Another case study looked at a 16-year-old male teenager with a five-week-old football injury who had daily headaches and "a sense of fogginess" (concentration difficulties). He reported significant improvement after the second visit, with near-complete symptom resolution after the fifth visit (within two weeks of care). After seven weeks of care, he successfully returned to normal activities, including playing football.

Dizziness and vertigo are also common residuals from concussion and were present in a 30-year-old woman just three days following a motor vehicle accident. She also complained of headache, neck pain, back pain, and numbness in both arms. The case study noted significant improvement after nine visits within an 18-day time frame.

What Can I Do to Stop a Migraine?

Migraines can be life-altering! They can stop us from being able to enjoy a child's piano recital, participate in family events, go to work, or simply do household chores! Wouldn't it be nice to have ways to self-manage these miserable, often disabling headaches? Here are some options!

1. RELAXATION THERAPY: Search for a calm environment, turn off the lights (photophobia, or light sensitivity, is a common migraine complaint), minimize sound/noise (due to "hyperacusis"), and sleep if possible. Monitor the room temperature and/or use

hot/cold compresses to the head and/or neck regions to relax tight muscles (heat) and reduce pain and swelling (cold). Similarly, a warm shower or bath can have similar beneficial effects.

2. SLEEP WELL: Migraines can interfere with falling asleep, they can wake you up during the night, and they are often triggered by NOT getting a good night's sleep. To improve your sleep quality: a) Establish regular sleeping hours. Wake up and go to bed at consistent times every day, including weekends. b) Keep daytime naps short (20-30 min. max). c) "Unwind" at the end of the day – try soothing music, a warm bath, or reading a favorite book (avoid suspenseful movies). d) Don't eat/drink too much before bedtime as heavy meals, caffeine, nicotine, and alcohol can interfere with sleep. e) Don't exercise intensely before bedtime (stretching is fine). f) Eliminate distractions in the bedroom, including TV and bringing work to bed. Close the bedroom door and use a fan to muffle out distracting noises. g) If you take any medications, check for known side effects, as many contain caffeine or other stimulants that can interfere with sleep – including some meds that treat migraines! Talk to your doctor and pharmacist!

3. EAT WELL: Be consistent about when you eat and don't skip meals (fasting increases the risk for migraine). Keep a food journal to figure out your migraine triggers and avoid foods that commonly trigger migraines like chocolate, aged cheeses, caffeine, and alcohol. Try eliminating these and see how you feel!

4. EXERCISE REGULARLY: This is MOST IMPORTANT for migraine management as it facilitates sleep cycles and stimulates the release of endorphins and enkephlins that help block pain. It also helps fight obesity, which is another risk factor for headaches.

Tension-Type Headaches – Management Strategies

Headaches (HA) can significantly alter a person's quality of life. Moreover, they can interfere and sometimes even prevent an individual from performing important activities such as going to work, attending school, or participating in group activities such as sports, music programs, holiday gatherings, and more. The focus of this month's Health Update is on Tension-Type Headaches (TTH), a common "primary headache" with tremendous socioeconomic impact.

Compared with migraine headaches, tension-type headaches are actually more common and can be equally as disabling. A recent study reviewing popular treatment approaches for TTH reported that establishing an accurate diagnosis is important prior to beginning treatment and finding "…non-drug management is crucial." Recommendations regarding treatment also include becoming educated about TTH, obtaining reassurance, and identifying trigger factors that can precipitate a TTH. Psychological treatments with scientifically-proven benefit include relaxation training, EMG biofeedback, and "cognitive-behavioral therapy" (CBT). Physical therapy, chiropractic, and acupuncture are widely used, but further research supporting these approaches is needed. The researchers state "simple analgesics" are the primary drug choice for TTH, but they strongly oppose the use of combination analgesics, triptans, muscle relaxants, and opioids, "….and it is crucial to avoid frequent and excessive use of simple analgesics to prevent the development of medication-overuse headache." They state that the tricyclic antidepressant amitriptyline is "drug of first choice" when treating chronic TTH, but they point out side effects can be significant, thus hampering their use. The researchers conclude that the treatment of frequent TTH is often difficult, and multidisciplinary approaches can be helpful. THIS IS WHERE CHIROPRACTIC FITS IN! These researchers state that non-drug approaches as well as medications "…with higher efficacy and fewer side effects [are] urgently needed." They advise that future studies need to focus on optimizing treatment programs to best suit the individual patient utilizing psychological, physical, and pharmacological-treatment approaches.

So, what can chiropractic bring to the table in this "team" treatment approach? First of all, it is non-drug oriented, the need of which clearly was emphasized in this study. Second, the presence of muscle tension at the base of the skull/top of the neck can be addressed VERY SPECIFICALLY with spinal manipulation of the cervical spine, active release, myofascial release, trigger point therapy, manual cervical traction, and more! Third, the use of NON-PRESCRIPTION nutrients such as ginger, tumeric, boswellia, Bromelain, white willow bark, fish oil/omega-3 fatty acids are all non-drug (with fewer potential side effects) options that facilitate in controlling inflammation. Using a home cervical traction device can also be VERY HELPFUL! Specific exercise training aimed at muscle relaxation, stretching, and strengthening (especially the deep neck flexors) can ALL BE MANAGED by a doctor of chiropractic!!!

Posture and Headaches

Headaches (HA) play a significant role in a person's quality of life and are one of the most common complaints that chiropractors see. This comes as no surprise, as one survey reported 16.6% of adults (18 years and older) suffered from migraines or other severe headaches during the last three months of 2011. Another study reported that head pain was the fifth LEADING CAUSE of emergency department (ED) visits in the United States and accounted for 1.2% of all outpatient visits. These statistics are even worse for females (18-44 years old), where the three month occurrence rate was 26.1% and the third leading cause for ED visits! Because of the significant potential side effects of medications, many headache sufferers turn to non-medication treatment approaches, of which chiropractic is one of the most commonly utilized forms of "complementary and alternative approaches" in the management of tension-type headaches. So, why are headaches so common? Let's talk about posture!

Posture plays a KEY ROLE in the onset and persistence of cervicogenic headaches. If there is such a thing as "perfect posture," it might "look" something like this: viewing a person from the front (starting at the feet), the feet would flair slightly outwards symmetrically, the medial longitudinal (inside) arch of the feet would allow enough space for an index finger to creep under to the first joint (and NOT flat like so many), the ankles would line up with the shin bones (and NOT roll inwards), the knees would slightly "knock" inwards and hips would line up squarely with the pelvis. The shoulders would be level, the arms would hang freely and not be pronated (rolled) inwards, and head would be level (not tilted). From the side view, the knees would not be hyperextended nor flexed, the shoulders would not be forward (protracted) and MOST IMPORTANT (at least for headaches), the head would NOT be forward and be able to have a perpendicular line drawn from the floor through the shoulder, as this line should pass through the outer opening of the ear. As the head "translates" or shifts forwards, for every inch of "anterior head translation" (AHT), it essentially gains 10 pounds in weight , which the upper back and neck muscles have to counter balance!

A leading University of California medical author, Dr. Rene Calliet, MD, wrote that this altered posture can add up to 30 pounds of abnormal weight to the neck and can "…pull the entire spine out of alignment." It can also reduce the lung's vital capacity by 30%, which can contribute to all sorts of breathing-impaired health problems! Think of carrying a 30-pound watermelon around your neck all day – the muscle pain from fatigue would be tremendous! If this is left uncorrected, chronic neck pain and headaches from pinching off the top three nerves in the neck is likely. The combination of AHT and shoulder protraction may also lead to the development of an upper thoracic "hump" and potentially into a "Dowager Hump" if the Midback vertebrae become compressed (wedged). An increased rate of mortality of 1.44 is reportedly associated with this faulty posture!

Between chiropractic adjustments, posture retraining exercises, other postural corrective care, and strength exercise training, we WILL help you correct your faulty posture so that neck pain and headaches STOP and don't progress into a chronic, permanent condition.
Headaches: How Does Chiropractic Help?

Headaches (HA) can be tremendously disabling, forcing sufferers away from work or play into a dark, quiet room to minimize any noise and light that intensifies the pain. According to the National Headache Foundation, there are over 45 million Americans who suffer from chronic, re-occurring headaches, of which 28 million are of the migraine variety. Also, approximately 20% of children and adolescents deal with headaches that can interfere significantly with their daily routines. There are many different types of headaches and many sub-types within the main categories. Here are a few: Tension HA (also, called cervicogenic HA), migraine, mixed headache syndrome (a mixture of migraine and tension HAs), cluster (less common but the most severe), sinus headaches, acute headaches, hormone headaches, chronic progressive headaches (traction or inflammatory HAs), and MANY more! Just "GOOGLE" "headache classification" for the daunting list! Let's take a look at how chiropractic manages these headaches!

According to a study completed in 2005, a review of the published literature revealed good evidence that intensity and frequency of HAs are indeed helped by chiropractic intervention. They limited their review to cervicogenic headaches and spinal manipulation and noted the need for larger scale studies. The well-respected Cochrane database reported spinal manipulation (SM) as an effective treatment option with short-term benefits similar to amitriptyline, a commonly prescribed medication for migraine HA patients.

For cervicogenic HA, the combination of neck exercises and SM was found to be effective in both the short- and long-term, and SM was superior to massage or placebo (sham or "fake" manipulation). Regarding the question of treatment frequency of SM plus up to two modalities (heat and soft tissue therapy), a preliminary study found that when comparing patients receiving one, three, or four visits per week for three weeks, those receiving 9-12 treatments during the three weeks had the most benefit. Regarding the questions, "what is affected by SM" and, "why does SM work" for cervicogenic HA patients, a study describes the intimate relationship between the upper cervical nerve roots (C1-3), the trigeminal (cranial nerve V), the spinal accessory (cranial nerve XI), and the vascular system. Inflammation within these structures and their relationship with the trapezius and SCM muscles help us understand the "why" and "how" of SM and referred pain pattern to the face and head in those with cervicogenic HAs. Realizing this is a bit "technical", feel free to GOOGLE these structures and you'll appreciate the close proximity they have to each other and how adjustments, or SM, applied to the upper cervical spine can affect this region. It has also been reported that SM and strengthening of the deep neck flexor muscles benefits the cervicogenic HA patient. Many HA sufferers have combinations of symptoms including dizziness, neck pain, concentration "fog", fatigue, and others, which were found to also respond to SM applied to the upper cervical spine. One study reported a 36% reduction in pain killer medication use in a group of cervicogenic headache patients receiving SM but no reduction in the patient group receiving soft-tissue therapy. The list of research studies goes on and on! So WHAT are you waiting for? TRY CHIROPRACTIC for your headache management!!!

Chiropractic and Sinus Headaches

Sinus **headaches** refer to pain in the head typically in and around the face. Most of us are knowledgeable about two of our four sinuses: the frontal (forehead) and maxillary (our "cheek bones"). The other two sinuses (called ethmoid and sphenoid) are much less understood. As chiropractors, many patients ask us about sinus problems, as all of us have had a stuffy nose due to a cold and have felt this pain in our face and head. Those of us who have suffered from sinus infections REALLY know how painful sinusitis can get! This month, let's take a look at our sinuses and what we can do to self-manage the problem.

First, an anatomy lesson... As stated above, there are four paired, or sets, of sinuses in our head: Maxillary: Pain/pressure in the cheekbones, sometimes referring pain to the teeth. These drain sideways (if you lay on your side, the side "up" drains down into the downside maxillary sinus and into the nose). Frontal:

Pain/pressure in the forehead. These drain downward (when we're upright, looking straight ahead). Ethmoidal: Pain/pressure between and/or behind the eyes. These drain when we lean forwards. Sphenoidal: Cause pain/pressure behind the eyes, top of the head and/or back of the head (which can be extreme). These drain best when lying face pointing down towards the floor, but they can be stubborn to drain!

Sinusitis, or rhinosinusitis, by definition is an inflammation of the sinus lining (mucous membrane) and is classified as follows: Acute – a new infection which can last up to four weeks and are divided into two types: severe and non-severe; Recurrent acute – four or more separate acute episodes within one year; Subacute – an infection lasting 4-12 weeks; Chronic infections lasting >12 weeks; and Acute exacerbation of chronic sinusitis – recurring bouts of chronic sinusitis.

One cause of sinusitis can include an "URI" (upper respiratory tract infections) most often in the form of a virus (such as rhinovirus — there are over 99 types have been identified, or better known as "the common cold"). Bacteria can also cause a sinus infection. These infections tend to last longer and can follow a viral infection. A third cause is a fungal infection. These are more common in diabetic and other immune deficient patients. Chemical irritants such as cigarette smoke and chlorine fumes can also trigger sinusitis. Chronic sinusitis can be caused by anything that irritates the sinuses for >12 weeks (viruses, bacteria, environmental irritants, tooth infections, and more). Allergies are also a common cause of sinusitis whether they are environmental and/or food/chemical induced.

Chiropractic care for sinusitis includes primarily symptomatic care with sinus drainage techniques such as facial and cranial bone manipulation/mobilization, lymphatic pump and drainage techniques, instruction in self-stretch of the sinuses (such as an outward pull of the cheek bones in different positions of the head), nutritional counseling (such as 1000mg of vitamin C every 2-4 hours) and anti-inflammatory herbs and vitamins (see prior

Health Updates), cervical and mid-back manipulation, training in nasal saline rinsing (Nasaline, Nettie Pot), moist heat (towels, steam), and of course, chicken soup! Co-management with your primary care doc may be needed at times, if medications are warranted.

How Does Chiropractic Help Headaches?

Headaches are one of the most common reasons people seek chiropractic care. Many patients with headaches benefit significantly from adjustments made to the upper cervical region. So, the question is, how does adjusting the neck help headaches? To help answer this question, let's look at a study that was recently published that examined this exact issue...

It's been said that if one understands anatomy, determining WHERE the problem is located becomes easy. So, let's take a look at the anatomy in the upper most part of the neck. In the study previously mentioned (http://www.ncbi.nlm.nih.gov/pubmed/21278628), the authors found an intimate relationship between the muscles that connect the upper 2 cervical vertebra (C1 and 2) together and their anatomical connection to the dura mater (the covering of the spinal cord). They identified this anatomical connection between the muscles that span between the back aspect of C1/2 and the dural connection as having a significant role in the development of headaches usually referred to as cervicogenic headaches.

There are several reasons why chiropractors adjust or manipulate the upper cervical vertebrae in patients with headaches. The obvious reason is simply because it helps to reduce the intensity, frequency and duration of headaches. The reason it works is this: If one or both of the upper 2 vertebrae (C1 and C2, also referred to as the atlas and axis, respectively) are either blocked or fixed and cannot properly move

20

independently, then there is an abnormal change in the biomechanics in that region. Similarly, if one of the two vertebrae is rotated or shifted in reference to the other, a similar biomechanical "lesion" or problem occurs (often referred to as a "subluxation"). You can take all the ibuprofen, Aleve, Tylenol or other perhaps stronger, prescription medication for the headache, but it is not logical that the biomechanical problem at C1 and/or C2 is going to change by inducing a chemical change (i.e., taking a pill). All you're doing is masking the symptoms for a while, at best.

Many people find that after a several chiropractic adjustments, their headaches are significantly improved. This is because restoring proper biomechanics to the C1/2 region reduces the abnormal forces on the vertebrae as well as any abnormal pull or traction of the posterior cervical muscles on the dural attachment. It has been reported that the function of this muscle/dura connection is to resist excessive movement of the dura towards the spinal cord when we look upwards and forwards. During neurosurgery, observation of mechanical stress on the dura was found to be associated in patients with headaches. In chronic headache sufferers, adjustments applied to this area results in significant improvement. There is no other treatment approach that matches the ability that adjustments or manipulation have in restoring the C1/2 biomechanical relationship thus, helping the headache sufferer. Another treatment option that has been shown to benefit the headache patient is injections to this same area. However, given the side effects of cortisone, botox, and other injectable chemicals, it's clear that chiropractic should be utilized first. It's the safest, most effective, and fastest way to restore function in the C1/2 area, thus relieving headaches.

Is it a Migraine?

There are MANY different types of **headaches**, of which migraines are a common type. This discussion will concentrate on some unique characteristics that are associated with migraine headaches. This information may help you understand what type of headache you're having. A unique feature of migraine headaches is that prior to the start of the headache, there is often a pre-headache "warning" that the migraine is about to commence. This is often referred to as an "aura," and it can vary from a few minutes to a few hours, or in some cases, two days prior to the start of the migraine. Here are some of the more common "warning signs" that you are having, or are about to have, a migraine:

• Neck pain. In an online survey, the National Headache Foundation found that 38% of migraine patients "always," and 31% "frequently" had neck pain accompany their migraine headache.

• Frequent urination. This can precede the migraine by an hour or as much as two days.

• Yawning. A 2006 article in the journal Cephalgia reported that about 36% of migraine sufferers describe yawning as a common pre-migraine warning. This can occur quite frequently, such as every few minutes.

• A "sensory aura" may occur on half of the body, moving from the finger tips through the arm, across the face, or elsewhere and usually includes a temporary lack of feeling as if the body region is "half asleep."

• Nausea and vomiting. This is a common aura. According to the American Migraine Study II (a mail survey of more than 3,700 migraine patients) 73% reported nausea and 29% vomiting. Another study reported that migraine sufferers who have nausea/vomiting usually have more severe migraine headaches and get less relief from migraine medications compared to those who do not get nausea or vomiting.

• Other common auras or "sensitivities" during the migraine include bright light, noise, and/or smells (like perfumes), and many migraine sufferers seek refuge in a dark, quiet room and try to sleep.

• Physical activity. Routine activities such as walking, climbing steps, running, weight lifting, or sexual activity can trigger a migraine and/or increase the intensity of an existing migraine headache.

• Trouble speaking. Difficulty "getting the words out" or formulating thought (staying on task) can be another warning sign of an impending migraine. Obviously, if this is the first time this symptom has occurred and it's "…out of the ordinary," we'll have to make sure it's not something more serious (…like a stroke)!

• Weakness. This may occur in an arm or leg or entire half of the body (left or right side) and also could be a more serious sign of a stroke, but it is also a fairly common pre-migraine aura.

• Visual aura. This can include double vision and / or vertigo (balance loss with a spinning feeling). This often occurs in a special type of migraine called a "basilar-type migraine" and symptoms can include dizziness, double vision or loss of vision. The balance loss is often associated with a "bad migraine" and occurs when the migraine is stronger or more intense than usual.

• "Headache hangover." This usually occurs after the migraine has passed and people describe a feeling of being "wiped out." Symptoms can include fatigue, difficulty concentrating, weakness, dizziness, lightheadedness, and extreme energy loss.

In many cases, adjustments applied to the neck and upper back, especially when delivered BEFORE the migraine, can reduce the intensity and in some cases STOP the migraine from even starting!

Do Chiropractors Help Patients With Headaches?

This seems like an easy question to answer, doesn't it? The answer of course being, YES!!! However, there are many people who suffer with **headaches** who have never been to a chiropractor or have not even ever considered it as a "good option."
So, rather than having me "reassure you" that chiropractic works GREAT for headache management, let's look at the scientific literature to see if "they" (the scientific community) agree or not.

In a 2011 meta-analysis, researchers reviewed journals published through 2009 and found 21 articles that met their inclusion criteria and used the results to develop treatment recommendations. Researchers discovered there is literature support utilizing Chiropractic care for the treatment of migraine headaches of either episodic or chronic migraine. Similarly, support for the Chiropractic treatment of cervicogenic headaches, or headaches arising from the neck region (see last month's Health Update), was reported. In addition, joint mobilization (the "non-cracking" type of neck treatment such as figure 8 stretching and manual traction) or strengthening of the deep neck flexor muscles may improve symptoms in those suffering from cervicogenic headaches as well. The literature review also found low load craniocervical mobilization may be helpful for longer term management of patients with episodic or chronic tension-type headaches where manipulation was found to be less effective.

Okay, we realize this is all fairly technical, so sorry about that. But, it is important to "hear" this so when people ask you why are going to a chiropractor for your headaches, you can say that not only that it helps a lot, but there are a lot of scientific studies that support it too!

Bottom line is that it DOES REALLY HELP and maybe, most importantly, it helps WITHOUT drugs and their related side effects. Just ask someone who has taken some of the headache medications what their side-effects were and you'll soon realize a non-drug approach should at least be tried first since it carries few to no side effects.

What Kind of Headache Do I Have?

Headaches come in MANY different sizes, shapes, and colors. In fact, if you search "headache classification," you will find the IHS (International Headache Society) 152 page manual (PDF) lists MANY different types of headaches! Last month, we discussed migraine headaches. This month, we'll talk about the other headache types. So WHY is this important? Very simply, if we know the type of headache you have, we will be able to provide you with the proper treatment. Headaches are classified into two main groups: "primary" and "secondary" headaches. The "Primary" headache list includes: 1) Migraine; 2) Tension-type; 3) Cluster; 4) "Other primary headaches," of which eight are listed. One might think that with this simple breakdown of the different types of headaches it should be easy to diagnose a type of headache. Unfortunately, that's NOT true! In fact, a 2004 study published that 80% of people with a recent history of either self or doctor diagnosed sinus headache had NO signs of sinus infection and actually met the criteria for migraine headaches! So, the more we can learn about the different types of headaches, the more likely that we will arrive at an accurate diagnosis.

Tension-Type Headaches : This is the most common type affecting between 30-78% of the general population. It is usually described as a constant ache or pressure either around the head, in the temples, or the back of the head and/or neck. There is typically NO nausea/vomiting, and tension-type headaches rarely stop you from performing normal activities. These headaches usually respond well to chiropractic adjustments and to over-the-counter medications like Advil, aspirin, Aleve, and/or

Tylenol, though we'd prefer you first reach for an anti-inflammatory herb like ginger, turmeric, bioflavonoid, and the like as these have less stomach, liver, and/or kidney related side-effects. These headaches are typically caused by contraction of the neck and scalp muscles, which can be result of stress, trauma, lack of sleep, eyestrain, and more.

Cluster Headaches : These are less common, typically affect men more than women, and occur in groups or cycles. These are VERY DISABLING and usually arise suddenly and create severe, debilitating pain usually on only one side of the head. Other characteristics include: a watery eye, sinus congestion, or runny nose on the same side of the face as the headache. An "attack" often includes restlessness and difficulty finding a pain-reducing, comfortable position. There is no known cause of cluster headaches, though a genetic or hereditary link has been proposed. The good news is that chiropractic adjustments can reduce the intensity, frequency, and duration of cluster headaches!

Sinus Headaches : Sinusitis (inflamed sinuses) can be due to allergies or an infection that results in a headache. This may or may not include a fever, but the main distinguishing feature here is pain over the infected sinus. There are four sets of sinuses. Many people know about the frontal (above the eyes on the forehead) and maxillary (under the eyes in our cheeks) but the two sinuses deep in head (ethmoid and sphenoid sinuses) are much less known or talked about. These two deep sinuses refer pain to the back of the head, and when infected, it feels like the back of the head could explode. Lying flat is too painful so sitting up is necessary. Chiropractic adjustments applied to the sinuses, upper neck, and lymphatic drainage techniques work GREAT in these cases!

Headaches, Neck Pain and Concussion

Have you ever "banged" your head from falling? For those playing backyard football, soccer, hockey, or baseball as kids or adults, it's really quite common. So, how can we tell when the "bang" is dangerous vs. not? And, how does a concussion occur?

What is a concussion? A concussion is "traumatic brain injury" (TBI) where the brain is "jarred" and literally bruises as a result of some sort of trauma (a "bang").

What causes a concussion? Causation is usually from some sort of trauma either by being hit by a moving object (like a ball), from hitting the head during a fall, and even without a direct strike if the head is violently moved back and forth (such as in a "whiplash" injury resulting from a car accident). When there is no direct strike of the head and in the absence of being "knocked out," the person may not be aware that they have a concussion.

What are the symptoms associated with concussion? Immediate symptoms usually include a **headache** and a reduced level of alertness or consciousness. A concussion temporarily interferes with the way the brain works and as a result (depending on the specific location and degree of the "brain bruise") it can affect memory (short term the greatest), levels of awareness, judgment, feeling "spacey," reflexes, speech, balance, coordination and sleep patterns. Other symptoms may include nausea and/or vomiting. Most people describe the experience as an abrupt injury where a bright flash of light occurs in the visual field that blocks the vision temporarily. Many do not actually become unconscious but may say they "blacked out" for a second or two. When unconsciousness does occur, the length of time they are "out" may be a way of determining severity. Symptoms can vary from mild to severe and the following are EMERGENCY symptoms where immediate health care provision is necessary: significant changes in alertness and consciousness, convulsions or seizures, muscle weakness on one or both sides, persistent confusion, persistent unconsciousness (coma), repeated vomiting, unequal pupils, unusual eye movements and walking problems. Neck injury is often associated with a head injury, which is why the injured person is stabilized on a board before being transported. Symptoms during recovery include being withdrawn, easily upset, confused, having a hard time with tasks that require memory and/or concentrating, having mild headaches and sensitivity to noise.

What tests are commonly performed on the post-concussive patient and, what is the treatment? A physical exam can include a careful evaluation of the cranial nerves such as pupil size and eye movement, as well as assessment of one's thinking ability, coordination and reflexes. Special tests may include an EEG (brain wave test), especially when seizures are involved. A head CT scan or head MRI. Treatment may require a hospital stay if severe signs are present. A "wait & watch" approach is often practiced but prompt gentle chiropractic approaches often facilitates healing and should strongly be considered. Refraining from rigorous sports is strongly advised.

Do Chronic Sinus Problems Cause Headaches?

Many of us have had sinus related **headaches**, right? You know, these are the headaches that hurt over the sinuses (above the eyes or in the cheek bones next to your nose) and, when you blow your nose, it's not pretty! Sinus infections often lead to sinus headaches – wouldn't you say that's a true statement?

A recent November 2011 study begs to differ. Researchers took 58 patients with a diagnosis of "sinus headache" made by their primary care physician and asked them the following questions:

1. Have you had a previous diagnosis of migraine or tension-type headache?

Is their clinical evidence of a sinus infection during the past 6 months?

- Is there the presence of "mucopurulent secretions" (that's the "not so pretty stuff" when we blow our nose)?All 58 patients clearly seemed to have chronic sinusitis with an acute flair up and were given complete thorough examinations by a neurologist and an ears, nose, throat specialist (otolaryngologist) on a monthly basis for 6 months during treatment. The surprising results showed that final diagnosis in these 58 cases were 68%, 27% and 5% of the patients really had migraine, tension-type headache and chronic sinusitis with recurrent acute episodes, respectively. Treatment during the 6 months included antibiotic therapy in 73% of the patients with tension-type headache and 66% with migraine. Sinus endoscopy (taking a look up the sinuses with a scope – ouch!) was performed in 26% of the patients, and therapeutic nasal septoplasty (surgery!) was performed in 16% of the migraine patients and 13% of patients with tension-type headache (a pretty BIG mistake, wouldn't you say?). The conclusion was that many patients with self-described or primary care physician diagnosed "sinus headaches" have no sinonasal abnormalities but instead, met the criteria for migraine or tension-type headache.So, what does this mean? Well, for one thing, too many antibiotics are prescribed for tension-type or migraine headaches and have no place in the treatment process of these two common headache categories. Side effects of antibiotics include (but are not limited to): stomach and intestinal irritation, nausea, and if one is allergic to the antibiotic, a potentially life-threatening condition call anaphylactic shock. Let's not forget to mention that sinus surgery was performed in 29% of the cases where the sinuses were NOT causing the headaches and we all know the risks of undergoing anesthesia and surgery can include death and infections, among other problems.Chiropractic was reported to be a wise choice in the treatment of headaches by several publications, one of which

29

provided a large review of the literature on the "Effectiveness of manual therapies: the UK evidence report," released in 2010 (http://chiromt.com/content/18/1/3). In this report, both migraine and cervicogenic-type (headaches that start in the neck) headaches were found to have strong research support for manipulation or, chiropractic adjustments. In this day and age, you can be very confident that choosing chiropractic services for headache treatment is a wise, safe, and very cost-effective approach for a very disabling condition.

Dangerous Headaches

This month's topic will address dangerous **headaches**. To keep this in perspective, most headaches are NOT dangerous. In fact, tension-type headaches and migraines are very common and remain the focus of most health care providers and patients who suffer from headaches. With that said, it's important to discuss the signs and symptoms that might help all of us differentiate between headaches that are safe versus those which are not safe.

The most important factor to consider is when the "typical" headache is suddenly "different." Some of these "different" symptoms may include slurred speech, difficulty communicating or formulating thought, seizures, fainting or loss of consciousness (even for a few seconds), memory lapses, double or blurred vision, profound dizziness, numbness in the face or half of the body, an "alarm" should sound off telling you to get this checked ASAP as these symptoms, when they deviate from "the norm" may be indicative of a more serious condition. This can be challenging as seizures are often related to migraines and might be a common symptom of a migraine headache for some migraine sufferers.

Signs of a dangerous headache include:

1. A headache that starts suddenly, especially if it's of a severe degree.
2. Headaches that start later in life, especially after the age of 50.
3. A change in the quality of headaches.
4. Visual changes, including double vision or loss of vision.
5. Weakness, numbness, or any other neurological symptoms.
6. Fevers – especially of rapid onset.
7. Change in mental status including sleepiness, hallucinations, speech changes or confusion.
8. Weight loss.

If there is ever ANY doubt about a dangerous headache, your physician should be contacted. Typically, the migraine patient will notice a fairly consistent set of symptoms and even though the headaches can vary in intensity, the sequence of events is fairly consistent. Dangerous headaches are the ones that deviate significantly from that migraine sufferer's "norm." For example, suppose a patient's "typical" migraine is: aura (bright, flashy lights in the visual field or, a strange odor precedes the migraine about 30 min. before the headache strikes), followed by a gradually increasing pain in half of the head which worsens to a point of nausea and sometimes vomiting if something isn't done to stop it (such as a chiropractic adjustment and/or some form of medication). If this is that patient's "usual," IF any of the 8 items previously listed above accompany the headache, it should be further evaluated – often requiring an EEG (electroencephalogram) and/or MRI (Magnetic Resonant Image). The EEG will test for any electrical signal changes in the brain and the MRI will show space occupying structures such as tumors, bleeding, infection, aneurism, and if performed with a contrast agents, arterial malformations (that is, abnormal networks of blood vessels).

Tension-Type Headaches

At some point, everyone will have a **headache**, whether it's caused by stress, lack of sleep, hormones, or even self-induced after having way too much fun the night before! For the most part, headaches are not indicative of a dangerous underlying condition, but they can be (…a topic for a future article). The focus of this article is to discuss the most common form of headache: the tension-type headache.

Tension-type headaches (TTHA) are defined by the Mayo Clinic as "a diffuse, mild to moderate pain that's often described as feeling like a tight band around your head." Ironically, even though this is the most common form of headache, the causes of TTHA are not well understood. These are sometimes described as muscle contraction headaches but many experts no longer think muscle contractions are the cause. They now feel that "mixed signals" coming from nerve pathways to the brain are to blame and may be the result of "overactive pain receptors."

Regardless of the cause, the triggers of tension headaches are well known and include stress, depression/anxiety, poor posture, faulty/awkward work station set-ups, jaw clenching, and many others. Risk factors for TTHA include being a woman (studies show that almost 90% of woman experience tension headaches at some point in life) and being middle aged (TTHAs appear to peak in our 40s, though they are not limited to any one age group). Complications associated with TTHAs may include job productivity loss, family and social interaction disruption, and relationship strain. The diagnosis is typically made by excluding other dangerous causes of headaches and when all the test results return "normal," the diagnosis of TTHA is made.

Strategies for managing TTHAs include:

- Heat and/or cold is often helpful as some patients prefer one over the other. Alternating between ice and heat is sometimes the most effective approach.

- Controlling stress by trimming out less important duties or "…taking on less" can help as well.
- Yoga, meditation, biofeedback and relaxation therapy.
- An "ergonomic" assessment of a workstation and how it "fits" the headache patient can also yield great results.
- Other highly effective therapies include acupuncture, massage therapy, behavior and/or cognitive therapy as well as of course, chiropractic!

Chiropractic is a GREAT choice compared to standard medical care, especially when side effects to medications exist. This is because manipulation of the cervical spine addresses the cause of the headache and doesn't just try to "cover up" the pain. In 2001, Duke University reported compelling evidence that spinal manipulation resulted in almost immediate improvement for those with headaches that originate in the neck with significantly fewer side effects and longer-lasting relief compared to commonly prescribed medication. Chiropractic treatment approaches include (partial list): spinal manipulation, trigger point therapy, mobilization techniques, exercise training, physical therapy modality use, dietary and supplementation education / advice, lifestyle coaching, and ergonomic assessments.

Headaches: Causes and Treatment

Few conditions leave their victims as miserable and agitated as **headaches**. There are many causes of headaches including stress, odors, bright lights, noise, fatigue, certain foods, hormonal shifts, allergies, as well as genetic predisposition. With all the possible causes of headaches, it's not surprising many people seek help from many different approaches such as conventional medical therapies like pharmaceuticals and injections. Others prefer a non-drug treatment approach such as chiropractic, massage therapy, acupuncture, and nutritional counseling.

Usually, there is not one specific cause of headaches so treatment can focus on various areas. For example, the muscles that attach to the base of the skull in the neck and upper back are often very short and tight, resulting in pressure or a squeezing effect on the surrounding nerves and blood vessels — resulting in headaches. Chiropractic treatment includes methods aimed at reducing the tightness found in the joints and muscles. One of these approaches is called spinal manipulation or "adjustments" where the joints in the neck are moved to restore motion and reduce joint fixations. By relaxing the muscles and tension between the joints, the nerves in the neck are less pressured which, in turn, can reduce headaches. The top three nerves that exit the upper neck travel into the head and are often the culprit behind the onset of headaches. The second nerve from the top is the one responsible for causing radiating pain over the top of the skull which communicates with other nerves sometimes causing the pain behind the eye felt by some headache sufferers.

Another chiropractic approach in the management of headaches includes soft tissue therapy where trigger points found in tight muscles are addressed through various forms of massage and mobilization methods. Manual traction of the head and neck can also be highly effective in reducing the tension found in patients with headaches. Exercises the patient can perform on his or her own can also be beneficial. Some of these, such as range of motion exercises with and without resistance (example: pushing your head into your hand during neck movements) and posture re-training (chin tucks – reducing the forward head position), help address the limited motion problems of the neck. Cervical (neck) traction performed by placing a rolled up towel placed behind the neck while lying on the back so that the head can hang off the side of the bed can also be very helpful.

Other treatment approaches that chiropractors utilize include stress management (such as biofeedback, relaxation instructions, meditation, visualization, and others), diet modifications (as certain foods can trigger headaches), nutritional supplementation (such as fish oil, Vit. D, feverfew and others), and sleep restoration.

Headaches – How Does Chiropractic Work?

Headaches are a common complaint at chiropractic clinics. There are many causes of headaches, some of which are "idiopathic" or unknown. Some headaches arise from "vascular" (blood vessels) causes such as migraine and cluster headaches. These often include nausea and/or vomiting and can be quite disabling and require rest in a dark, quiet place sometimes for a half or a whole day. Another type of headaches can be categorized as "tension" headaches. These usually result from tightness in the muscles in the neck and upper back caused from stress, work, lack of sleep, sinusitis, and trauma (such as whiplash). So, "how does chiropractic work?" To answer this, let's first discuss what a doctor of chiropractic does when someone with headaches presents for care.

First, the history is very important! Here, a doctor of chiropractic will ask about how/when the headaches started. This may glean the actual cause of headaches such as a car accident or injury of some sort.

Next, they'll ask about activities that increase or create the headache, which gives them ideas of how they might help manage the headache patient. For example, when certain activities precipitate the onset of a headache, the doctor will offer assistance in how to modify the workstation and/or give specific exercises on a regular schedule to keep neck tension under control.

With information gathered about what decreases or helps relieve neck pain and headaches, a chiropractor will recommend treatments that can be done at home such as a home traction unit. This would be suggested if the patient reports "...pulling on my neck feels great!"

The quality of pain (throbbing = vascular, ache and tightness = neck), intensity of pain (0-10 pain scale), and timing (worse in the morning vs. evening) help them track change after treatment is rendered, usually gathered once a month.

The examination includes measuring the patient's blood pressure which can in itself create headaches when high, looking in the eyes to view the blood vessels in the back of the eye to make sure there is no evidence of increased pressure against the brain, ears – to see if there is an infection or wax blockage. This can help if there is dizziness and/or balance loss. The doctor of chiropractic will sometimes listen to the throat as well as the heart to see if there may be a blockage, a valve problem, or other issues.

Neck muscle tightness (spasm) will be evaluated along with the range of motion, paying particular attention to the positions/directions that increases and decreases pain, especially those that decrease pain.

Nerve function will be observed by checking reflexes, sensation, and muscle strength as well as correlating information like positions that decrease arm or leg pain will be included as any position that reduces pain in the arm or leg must be incorporated into an exercise.

X-rays may include bending "stress" views so that ligaments (that hold bones together) can be evaluated for "laxity" (torn and unstable). When this is found, the doctor may avoid adjustments to these vertebrae.

As you can see, if is very important do a thorough evaluation so headache patients can be properly managed. Treatment approaches include: 1. Adjustments; 2. Soft tissue therapy (trigger point stimulation, myofascial release); 3. Posture correction exercises and other exercises; 4. Education about job modifications; and 5. Co-management with other healthcare providers, if medication or injection therapy is needed.

Headaches – What Can YOU Do?

Headaches are one of the most common complaints for which patients seek chiropractic care. Chiropractic is especially helpful in the treatment of headaches because the three nerves that exit the top of the spine (upper neck) are often the cause of or directly related to headaches. These three nerves travel into the head and have to pass through a very thick group of muscles in the upper part of the neck near where these muscles attach to the base of the skull. This is why when you have headaches and rub the back of the neck, the muscles may feel tight and or tender. In fact, if enough pressure is applied over one of these three nerves, pain will radiate into the head following the course of the nerve, sometimes all the way into the eyes. When chiropractic treatment is applied in the upper neck region, it can reduce a headache and accompanying neck pain because the muscle tension is decreased and joint motion is restored.

The International Headache Society (IHS) has classified headaches into two main categories: primary and secondary. Primary headaches occur for no known reason and there are four groups of these:

1. migraine
2. tension-type
3. cluster
4. "other" primary headaches.

Secondary headaches are those with a specific cause such as sinus/allergy headaches, those associated with eye strain, a known medical condition, or those due to cold or flu. Both migraine and cluster headaches are "vascular" (related to the blood vessels expanding inside the head), resulting in a unique set of symptoms that includes nausea, vomiting, and pounding/throbbing, which can be quite debilitating.

The most common type is the tension-type of headache. A thorough history is necessary because there is no specific diagnostic test (lab or blood test) for tension-type headaches. Hence, the concept is to make sure the headache is not related to some other condition that is diagnosable by a blood or lab test and if present, having that condition properly managed. So, assuming all the tests come back "normal" and all other causes have been eliminated or "ruled out," the most common type of tension-type headache is "episodic," meaning they occur off and on, lasting minutes to days. The pain is usually described as, "…my whole head hurts." There is typically tightness or tension (NOT throbbing) described in the neck muscles and the intensity ranges from mild to moderate, not usually severe, where laying down is needed. Physical activity does not usually make it worse and there is no sickness to the stomach (nausea/vomiting), and no intense reaction to bright lights or noise (like there is with migraine & cluster types of headaches). There are sub-types of tension headaches that can occur simultaneous with migraines headaches, but the classic "aura" (a before the headache warning associated with migraine headaches) is usually not present.

Chiropractic treatment typically includes manipulation and mobilization of the neck, muscle release techniques, physical therapy modalities like electric stimulation, ultrasound, and others, exercise, stress and diet/nutritional management.

Headache – What Is It and What Can I Do About It?

"I woke up this morning with an excruciating headache. I thought the top of my head was going to blow off!"

"I notice as the day goes on, tightness in my neck worsens and I get a headache usually by 2-3pm."

"I don't know if I can do my work with my headaches."

Statements like these are common on case history forms patients fill out when they seek chiropractic care for their **headaches**. Many patients ask, "…what is a headache?" The National Institutes of Health (NIH) describe four types of headache: vascular, muscular contraction or tension, traction, and inflammatory.

The most common form of vascular headache is the migraine. Migraine sufferers usually complain of severe pain on one or both sides of the head, nausea or vomiting, and sometimes visual changes. There is often a heightened sensitivity to light or noise prompting migraine sufferers to lay in a dark, quiet room until the migraine passes. Women are more likely to suffer from migraines than men and the severity of symptoms can be so extreme that all activity must be stopped until it passes.

The next most common type of vascular headache is the toxic headache produced by a fever. Other vascular headache types include "cluster" headaches, which are characterized by repeated episodes of intense pain that start in one spot and spread out. These may only last a few minutes to an hour but carry a very high level of pain and activity intolerance. Another common type of vascular headache is that resulting from high blood pressure.

Muscle contraction or tension headaches involve tightening of the facial and neck muscles. These often start in the neck and radiate over the top or to the sides of the head. The muscles in the neck are usually extremely tight and tender and often, moderate pressure applied with the finger or thumb to these muscles will prompt radiating pain into and/or over the top of the head. This can also result in significant activity intolerance but usually not as severe as migraine or cluster headaches.

Traction and inflammatory headaches result because of other conditions that range from a sinus infection to a stroke. These types of headaches can serve as a warning sign of a more significant or serious condition. Another example is meningitis as well as other conditions affecting the sinuses, spine, neck, ear, and teeth.

The NIH suggests, when headaches occur three or more times a month, that "... preventive treatment is usually recommended." Certainly, in some cases, medication may be indicated but only after ruling out a more serious condition and after exhausting less invasive treatments that carry fewer side effects.

The American Chiropractic Association recommends:

1. Avoid long time periods of staying in one position (computer, sewing machine, reading, etc.) and take stretching/neck range of motion exercise breaks every ½ to 1 hour;
2. Exercise – walking, low impact aerobics;
3. Avoid teeth clenching (due to straining the temporomandibular – TMJ, or jaw joint);
4. Drink lots of water – stay hydrated.

Chiropractic care may include spinal manipulation (adjustments), nutritional advice (dietary suggestions, vitamin/mineral options such as a B complex), exercise, posture retraining, and relaxation techniques.

The Neck and Headache Connection

Patients with **headaches** also commonly complain of **neck pain**. This relationship is the rule, not the exception and therefore, treatment for headaches must include treatment of the neck to achieve optimum results. The term, "cervicogenic headaches" has been an accepted term because of the intimate connection between the neck and head for many years. There are many anatomical reasons why neck problems result in headaches. Some of these include:

- The first 3 nerves exiting the spine in the upper neck go directly into the head. They penetrate the muscles at the top of the neck near the attachments to the skull and therefore, any excess pressure on these nerves by the muscles or spinal joints will result in irritation and subsequent pain.
- The origin or nucleus of the 5th cranial nerve called the Trigeminal, innervates the sensation to the face and is located in the upper cervical region near the origin of the 2nd cervical spinal nerve, which innervates sensation to the back of the head up to the top. Therefore, problems located in the upper neck will often result in pain radiating up from the base of the skull/upper neck over the top of the skull to the eyes and /or face.
- The 11th cranial nerve that innervates the upper shoulders and muscles in the front of the neck arises from the top 5 to 7 spinal cord levels in the neck. Injury anywhere in the neck can result in spasm and pain in these large muscle groups.
- Other interconnections between the 2nd cervical nerve and trigeminal/5th cranial nerve include communication with the 7th cranial / facial nerve, the 9th cranial / glossopharyngeal nerve, and the 10th cranial / vagus nerve. These connections can affect facial muscle strength/movements, taste, tongue and throat movements, and stomach complaints such as nausea from these three cranial nerve interconnections, respectively.

When patients seek treatment for their headaches, a thorough examination of the neck, upper back, and cranial nerves is routinely performed for the above reasons. It is common to find upper cervical movement and vertebral alignment problems present in patients complaining of headaches. Tender points located between the shoulder blades, along the upper shoulders, on the sides of the neck and particularly, at the base of the skull are commonly found. Pain often radiates from the tender point over the top of the skull when pressure is applied in the upper neck/base of the skull area. Tenderness on the sides of the head, in the temples, over the eyes, and near the jaw joint are also common. Traction or pulling the head to stretch the neck is often quite pain relieving and this is often performed as part of the chiropractic visit and can also be applied at home with the use of a home cervical traction unit. Chiropractic adjustments applied to the fixated or misaligned vertebra in the upper neck often brings very satisfying relief to the headache sufferer. Exercises that promote movement in the neck, as well as strengthening exercises are also helpful in both reducing headache pain and in preventing occurrences, especially with stress or tension headaches.

Self-Management Approaches For Your Headache?

One of the reported causes of both migraine and tension **headache** is cervical muscle tension and spinal joint abnormalities in the neck. When considering treatment for headaches, whether it's a tension-type or migraine, there are many choices available. The question is, which of the many options offer the best benefit?

One study compared the effectiveness of physical therapy (PT) to that of relaxation and thermal biofeedback (RTB). Both groups were treated using one of these approaches, and if at least a 50% improvement was not achieved, the other form of treatment was then utilized. Results were calculated at 3, 6, and 12-month timeframes. The PT group was treated with standard physical therapy approaches that included:

- Posture correction for alignment of head and spine
- Cervical range of motion for neck and shoulders
- Isometric strengthening of the neck
- Flare-up management techniques
- Active self mobilization of the spine
- Whole body stretching

The goal was to target muscular abnormalities and those in this group were to perform the above twice per day for 30 min. The RTB group were instructed in relaxation and thermal biofeedback (RTB) treatment that focused on muscle relaxation, breathing exercises, and the use of a thermal feedback device that determines when the subject's temperature changes telling them if they are successfully relaxing. The participants were to practice at home and utilized audiotapes for relaxation and monitor success with the portable biofeedback unit.

Using the PT approaches, only 13% reported a successful outcome compared with 51% in the RTB group. In the follow-up at 3, 6 and 12 months, both groups reported continued benefit. When the subjects reported less than 50% benefit with either method, they were given the other treatment option, and the PT approach achieved a 47% success rate and the RTB 50%. These findings suggest that treatments that focus on muscle tension reduction (such as the RTB group) might result in a better outcome compared to only addressing posture, range of motion, and flexibility. However, as illustrated in the follow-up group, PT did have a positive beneficial effect. An important point – the subjects in the RTB group demonstrated the ability to reduce migraine pain and the associated disability by using a self-applied form of care. When teaching the patient to self-manage their condition by instruction and training, the greater the likelihood for a successful outcome.

Chiropractic focuses on many self-management training procedures including (but not limited to) the training of the use of ice vs. heat, exercises, proper methods of bending and lifting, as well as posture and strength. The use and instruction of relaxation is also a commonly recommended form of care, which this study found to be most beneficial.

Headaches: A Self-Assessment of Function

Headaches are a very common problem seen in chiropractic offices. They can vary from mild and barely noticeable to extreme, so much so that it results in total disability where a sufferer is restricted to bed rest in a dark, quiet room.

One inexpensive, reliable method to track a patient's progress is a self-administered test called the "Headache Disability Index" (HDI). This is a 25-question form that the headache sufferer completes and a total score is calculated. In the list of 25 questions, there are three choices for scoring: a "YES" response = 4 points, a "SOMETIMES" response = 2 points, and a "NO" response is not worth any points. The highest possible score = 100 (4 points x 25 questions). When patients present for chiropractic treatment, this method of assessment is often utilized and can be very helpful to determine the effectiveness of the care being provided, especially because of the lack of special assessments that exists for most types of headaches. Here is a list of questions that are included in the HDI:

- E1. Because of my headaches I feel handicapped.
- F2. Because of my headaches I feel restricted in performing my routine daily activities.
- E3. No one understands the effect my headaches have on my life.
- F4. I restrict my recreational activities (e.g. sports, hobbies) because of my headaches.
- E5. My headaches make me angry.
- E6. Sometimes I feel that I am going to lose control because of my headaches.
- F7. Because of my headaches I am less likely to socialize.
- E8. My spouse (significant other), or family and friends have no idea what I am going through because of my headaches.
- E9. My headaches are so bad that I feel I am going to go insane.

- E10. My outlook on the world is affected by my headaches.
- E11. I am afraid to go outside when I feel that a headache is starting.
- E12. I feel desperate because of my headaches.
- F13. I am concerned that I am paying penalties at work or at home because of my headaches.
- E14. My headaches place stress on my relationships with family or friends.
- F15. I avoid being around people when I have a headache.
- F16. I believe my headaches are making it difficult for me to achieve my goals in life.
- F17. I am unable to think clearly because of my headaches.
- F18. I get tense (e.g. muscle tension) because of my headaches.
- F19. I do not enjoy social gatherings because of my headaches.
- E20. I feel irritable because of my headaches.
- F21. I avoid traveling because of my headaches.
- E22. My headaches make me feel confused.
- E23. My headaches make me feel frustrated.
- F24. I find it difficult to read because of my headaches.
- F25. I find it difficult to focus my attention away from my headaches and on other things.

Some Headache Causes and Solutions

There are many people who frequently suffer from **headaches**, some even on a daily basis. Many feel this is "normal." In fact, when they visit a chiropractor for the first time for what they believe to be an unrelated issue, they may not even bring it up. They may only discuss it after being asked if they have headaches, as if everyone has headaches.

That's why it is very important to take a very thorough health and family history when a patient first presents for care at any doctor's office.

In this process, patients may offer clues to the cause of their headaches. For example, if a patients indicates that she has had headaches as long as she could remember and her family history includes her mother having headaches that were debilitating and an MRI revealed that part of her brain stem extended down into the upper part of the neck, this would prompt an MRI of the patient which could reveal a similar finding. Another example is a patient with headaches that occur one week prior to menstruation. This may lead to the trial of several nutritional vitamin / herbal approaches aimed at reducing fluid retention or build up that frequently occurs pre-menses. Other causes have included traumas from car accidents, slips and falls, and sports injuries. In these cases, the physical examination may lead to a diagnosis of abnormal biomechanics in the cervical spine and chiropractic treatment addressing these findings may prove very satisfying. Other causes may include stress and/or psychological conditions that required co-management with a mental health practitioner and/or the patient's primary care physician. The combined efforts of medication and chiropractic treatments are most satisfying for these patients.

In general, the cause of headaches are usually multi-factorial and therefore, the most effective treatment is a multi-dimensional approach in which chiropractic treatment methods are, in most cases, the most important contribution to the successful management of headaches. Chiropractic treatment approaches include spinal manipulation, mobilization, muscle release techniques such as trigger point therapy, longitudinal and /or transverse friction massage, massage therapy, manual and/or instrumental traction both at home and office, physical therapy modalities including ice/heat, electrical stimulation (several types), ultrasound, light/low level laser therapy, infrared, diet and nutritional counseling, and stress management. Co-management needed for some patients can be arranged through by their doctor of chiropractic and may include primary care physicians, physical medicine and rehabilitation physicians, pain management doctors, rheumatologists, internists, neurologists, physical therapists, as well as acupuncturists.

Headaches and Posture

Have you ever glanced at your reflection in a storefront window or mirror as you walked by and noticed your posture? Scary, isn't it? We all know that we should stand up straight, but we soon forget when as we fall back into our daily routine.

Poor posture is often due to years of standing slouched, a bad "habit" that usually starts at a young age. Just look around the next time you're in an airport or at a shopping mall and notice how many people have poor posture. In fact, a person's posture may reflect their present attitude and reveal if they're happy, sad, or depressed. Poor posture may be related to self-consciousness, especially during adolescence. It may also have a genetic component, as we frequently see a "trait" throughout family members with similar postural tendencies.

The most common postural fault associated with headaches is the forward-based head and shoulders. From the side, it appears that the head is significantly forward relative to the shoulders, the upper back is rounded forwards, and the shoulders are rolled forwards and rotated inward. One exercise that helps reduce this

47

postural bad habit is tucking in the chin and pretending a book is balancing on top of the head. The objective is to not allow the book to slide forward off your head and land on your toes!

It takes approximately three months of CONSTANT self-reminding before the new "good habit" posture becomes automatic, so be patient. Soon you'll "catch yourself doing it right" without thinking about it.

Frequently, posture is faulty lower down the "kinetic chain." The first link of the chain is the feet and the last link is the head. Since we stand on two feet, any change in that first link or the feet, can alter the rest of the chain, especially areas further away like the head, resulting in headaches. For example, if one leg is short, the pelvis drops, the spine shifts (scoliosis), the shoulder drops and the head shifts in an attempt to keep the eyes level. A short leg usually needs to be managed with a heel lift, an arch support, or combination of both to properly treat the headache patient.

Headaches and Management Options

Headaches are one of the more common conditions that enter the offices of primary care doctors, including chiropractors. The standard medical treatment revolves around the use of medications and/or injections. The standard chiropractic treatment approach includes manual therapies that may include spinal manipulation or adjustments, manual or mechanical cervical traction, mobilization techniques, trigger point therapy, nutritional counseling, and physical agents or modalities such as electrical stimulation, ultrasound, etc. While both approaches have their pros and cons, there are far fewer side effects associated with the chiropractic treatment option.

Headaches can generally be classified as primary or secondary. Primary Headaches include Migraine, Tension, and Cluster. Secondary headaches occur because another condition or injury is present such as after a car accident or slip and fall injury, an infection, a vascular injury—such as stroke, a medication side effect, psychiatric disorder, and/or a sinus, jaw, or dental condition.

When considering the use of complementary and alternative approaches available to patients with chronic tension-type headaches, a 2008 report revealed that 40% of 110 patients surveyed utilized some form of an alternative/complementary medical approach. The most frequently utilized was chiropractic (21.9%), followed by acupuncture (17.8%), and massage therapy (17.8%).

If you find yourself frequently utilizing over-the-counter medications such as an non-steroidal anti-inflammatory drugs (NSAIDs), it is probable that the chiropractic management approach will benefit your headache condition.

Frequently, in patients with headaches, the vertebrae in the upper neck lose their normal range of motion and the muscles in that region that attach to the base of the skull become overly tight and squeeze or compress the nerves that feed into the head. This results in radiating pain over the top or around the head, sometimes into the eyes. Chiropractic care can make it easier for you to move your head and neck forwards, back, rotate or twist, and side bend. This in turn reduces muscle tension and nerve pinching that may be present, which reduces headache pain.

Stress and Headaches

How does stress affect your well-being and how is stress related to getting headaches? Let's discuss the most common ways stress can make you more headache prone...

While most of us do not get enough sound, restful, and restorative sleep as it is, stress can interfere affect both the quantity and quality of sleep we do get. If you're tossing and turning all night, your body won't have the opportunity to refresh itself and this can add tension to your morning. If you then consume a lot of caffeine to help get you through the day, it can lead to a vicious cycle by hindering your ability to sleep the following night.

How we react to stress also affects us. Some of us literally "take it out' on our bodies, channeling the stress into our neck and shoulders. This can cause tension-type headaches where the muscles of your at the back of your neck become tight. "Knots" can develop in the muscles, sending shooting pains into your head.

Stress can affect us by disrupting our normal healthy routine. Instead of eating right and exercising, we resort to eating junk foods and avoiding the gym. Over-eating and not maintaining a healthy weight can add to the stress on the body, the spine, and the heart. Studies have shown that the risk for headaches is higher among those who are overweight or obese.

A lot of us think we handle stress well and just need a two-week vacation to get back on track. But really, two weeks off does little to change your life for the other fifty weeks during the year. The key is to learn how to handle and deal with stressors on a "day to day" basis. The presence of back pain or neck pain can also add stress to your life by making your everyday activities more difficult. If that's you, please see your doctor of chiropractic.

Since the presence of stress can increase your risk of headaches, becoming better at managing your stress levels can also help lower your risk. Each day, try to do something positive for yourself, and resist the temptation to worry about the future and fret about the past. Take each day as it comes and try to have positive thoughts. These practices can help improve your outlook and perspective. Try a different attitude in approaching the stressful things in your life. Sometimes just getting things into perspective and not stressing the small stuff are important to leading a more stress-free life, and enjoying the hidden pleasures that life brings to us each and every day.

Different Headaches and Chiropractic Care

Adults may experience many different kinds of headaches. A primary headache is a headache that is not a part of another disease process. Secondary headaches can come from a poor eyeglass prescription, diabetes, the flu, or even a brain tumor. The most common primary headaches are tension-type, migraine, and cervicogenic (from the neck).

Tension type headaches feel like a tight band around your head. Stress seems to aggravate them and women tend to get this type of headache more frequently. Females are also more affected by migraine headaches.

There are two types of migraine: classical and common. The classical migraine headache may start with nausea or sickness in the stomach and proceed to an intense throbbing pain on one side of the head. The common migraine lacks this nausea and is more common than the classical type.

In cervicogenic headache, neck function is prominently disturbed. In addition to neck pain, there are usually tight neck and shoulder muscles, and a limited range of motion.

Recent research has shown that the three above described headaches can also overlap with one another. In chiropractic, we look to the spine as an often-overlooked factor in headache treatment. By objectively analyzing spine function, the doctor will identify the joints that are restricted in their range of motion or show abnormal posture and alignment. Many patients on x-ray, or through external postural analysis from the side, can show forward head posture. This is where the neck seems to arise from the front of the chest rather than back over your shoulders.

The head is very heavy and with this poor posture, the muscles at the back of the neck must contract to restrain this heavy load.

There isn't one particular bone that is treated for these different types of headaches, the premise being that the headache is a symptom of another problem in the spine.

Chiropractic care has an excellent safety profile and several studies have shown that patents with headaches positively respond to chiropractic care without the side effects often seen with drug treatments. Chiropractic care is one of the most researched non-drug options available for patients. Unfortunately, many patients choose over-the-counter and prescription medications and don't consider more natural approaches that may get at the cause of the condition rather than just its effects.

How Can Exercise Help Your Headache?

For many patients with health conditions, exercise seems to be the furthest thing from their mind. For migraine sufferers, exercise itself can initiate a headache episode. And if you already have a headache, just the idea of going for a three-mile run will likely increase your pain, not lessen it.

But exercise is an integral component to overall health and that includes people who suffer from headaches too.

The key is to exercise when you are headache-free, to manage your exercises so that your spine is not excessively stressed, and make sure you have good flexibility of your spine before you begin loading it with exercises.

This is where chiropractic enters the picture. Your spinal flexibility is integral to maintaining good posture and assuring nerve impulses transmit freely from your brain to distant areas of the body. If you have a spinal problem, this may interrupt the free transmission of nerve impulses and make you susceptible to headache.

You may want to consider getting adjusted before strenuous exercise to make sure you have good spinal flexibility. After performing a strenuous activity, it may also be a good time to have your spine checked. Little by little, your spinal muscles will regain strength and you may find your headaches become a less dominate part of your life.

Other points to consider are getting adequate rest/sleep and to avoid overtraining because sleep deprivation can provoke a headache. You will also need to pay attention to water intake. Being dehydrated may also be a trigger for people with headaches. The bottom line is this: if you get the spinal care you need, if you watch strenuous movements that strain the spine, and if you get adequate rest and sleep, then you can begin exercising again despite your chronic headaches. Many patients with headaches say that stress is a trigger for their pain. Regular exercise can be a great way to deal with the stresses of life. Exercise is also key to your maintaining a healthy weight.

Are Headaches Undertreated?

With all the different types of pain relievers available at the corner drug store, you'd think headache sufferers would have a solution to their problem. However, such is not the case and headaches continue to be a great burden on society. What's more, it seems many doctors may even under-diagnose this common problem.

A 2008 study published in the British Journal of General Practice highlighted this widespread issue. The researchers studied over 91,000 adult patients who had recently reported a headache to their doctor. Amazingly, seventy percent of these patients were not given a diagnosis. It was suggested by the authors of the study that general medical physicians have difficulty in diagnosing headache presentations.

The spine is often overlooked as having the potential for causing a headache. Too often, headaches are thought to have their cause in the head. While this is where the pain is most prominent (as opposed to the neck), neck symptoms such as muscle tension, knots, and painful tissues also contribute to the pain picture. If your neck mobility is impaired, this can also be a indicator that the neck could be the source of your head pain. Sprains of the small vertebral joints can be enough to produce head pain and need to be addressed.

When the headache is thought to originate in the neck, it is called "cervicogenic."

Neck problems have also been implicated in certain cases of tension-type, as well as migraine headaches, but how this occurs exactly is still being investigated.

Whatever their cause, headaches have a devastating impact on our quality of life and need to be effectively treated. Chiropractic care has been shown in several studies to reduce headache pain and is an important non-drug option for patients.

Headaches From The Neck?

Cervicogenic headache is the term used to describe a headache that is caused by dysfunction in the neck. Overall, between 14-17.8% of patients with frequent headaches are believed to suffer from headaches of this nature.

The following is a list of clinical characteristics common among those struggling with cervicogenic headaches:

Unilateral (one-sided) head or face pain (rarely is it on both sides).

1. Pain is localized or stays in one spot, usually the back of the head, frontal, temporal (side), or orbital (eye) regions.
2. Moderate-to-severe pain intensity.
3. Intermittent attacks of pain that can last for hours or even days.
4. Pain is usually deep and non-throbbing, unless migraines occur at the same time.
5. Head pain is triggered by neck movement, sustained awkward head postures, applying deep pressure to the base of the skull or upper neck region, and/or taking a deep breath, cough or sneeze can trigger head pain.
6. Limited neck motion with stiffness.

A 2007 study (Funct Neurol 2007;22:145; Drottning M, Staff PH, Sjaastad O) looked at causes of cervicogenic headaches, specifically whiplash injuries of the neck. In this study, 587 whiplash patients were followed over a six-year period. About 8% of the whiplash sufferers developed a cervicogenic headache within six weeks of the initial trauma. Thirty-five percent of these patients were still suffering six years later. For a detailed discussion about how whiplash trauma can result in cervicogenic headaches, see **Whiplash Injury and Cervicogenic Headache**.

If you suffer from headaches and believe yours may originate from a musculoskeletal issue in your neck, a doctor of chiropractic can perform a comprehensive examination of your spine to see if sprains are present in either your cervical or thoracic joints and he or she will also review whether you've suffered a past trauma that could have affected the posture and mobility of these delicate spinal structures.

Headache and High Blood Pressure: A New Link?

Headaches are one of the common health complaints for which people seek out treatment. High blood pressure is also very common, affecting about 50 million Americans. Could the two be linked? Yes, but not in the way you may think. While some doctors question whether taking pain pills actually corrects the cause of the headache, there are also other perhaps more seemingly silent concerns. Is simply cutting the fire alarm when the house is on fire ever a good idea? If your headache is coming from a problem such as a joint dysfunction in the neck, is taking a pill going to do anything to help the joint injury?

We all see the TV commercials and the long pill aisles at the supermarket. Could our excessive use of these drugs be causing another problem, one that may not be explained on the pill bottle label?

Researchers looked at over-the-counter medications such as acetaminophen (e.g. Tylenol) and ibuprofen (e.g. Advil) to see if taking them over the long-term elevates an individual's risk for developing high blood pressure (Hypertension 2005;46:500. Women's Health Study I and II). The study investigated 5,123 women between the ages of 34 and 77 and followed them over many years.

Compared with women who did not use acetaminophen, the relative risk of high blood pressure for those who took >500 mg per day was 1.93 among older women and 1.99 among younger women. A relative risk of 1.93 is a 93% increase in risk.

For nonsteroidal anti-inflammatory drugs (e.g. ibuprofen), the risk of developing high blood pressure in older women also increased, ranging from a 78% to a 161% elevation. For younger women, the increased risks for hypertension ranged from a 10% increase to a 132% increase.

The authors of the study concluded that because acetaminophen and other nonsteroidal anti-inflammatory drugs are commonly used, they might contribute to the increased prevalence of high blood pressure in the United States.

Headaches Are Letting You Know...

...there is a problem. Our bodies often let us know there is something not quite right, but are we listening? Too often in life, with hectic day-to-day schedules, getting the kids to school and so on, we cannot be troubled by these little warning signs. So we often just take a pill to mask the pain and get on with our lives. But is this the best way to react to a warning signal?

If the smoke alarm shrilled in your home, what would you do? I hope you would get out as quickly as possible and call 911. Would you say to yourself, "maybe it will go away?" I hope not. And if there were a fire, would stopping the alarm help put out a raging inferno? Most likely, this will help things very little.

What if the alarm started to give little beeps (letting you know to change the battery). Would you change it with a fresh one or just remove it from the device?

I think most homeowners know the answers to these simple questions. And you would think that we would give the same correct concern when are bodies give us warning signals.

Unfortunately we often pay more attention to warning signs from our homes and automobiles (like that little clicking sound), than the most important house of all-our bodies.

When your neck muscles ache, this is a signal. When you turn your head and hear clicking sounds, this is another signal. And when a headache occurs, the signal is getting louder and louder. But are we listening?

It's better to think of these signals as just that, signals- not the actual problem. So when you take a drug to stop the signal, rarely is the actual problem being addressed.

So how are your signals and alarms?

Do you seem to take medications on a weekly or daily basis? A headache pill here and there is rarely an issue. But incorporating pain pills as part of your daily diet may be a health concern. They are not considered one of the five basic food groups. Side effects from these types of medications are rare, but the risks do increase with long-term use. Do you go through a small bottle each month?

A Deeper Look into Headaches

Headaches are REALLY common! In fact, two out of three children will have a headache by the time they are fifteen years old, and more than 90% of adults will experience a headache at some point in their life. It appears safe to say that almost ALL of us will have firsthand knowledge of what a headache is like sooner or later!

Certain types of headaches run in families (due to genetics), and headaches can occur during different stages of life. Some have a consistent pattern, while others do not. To make this even more complicated, it's not uncommon to have more than one type of headache at the same time!

Headaches can vary in frequency and intensity, as some people can have several headaches in one day that come and go, while others have multiple headaches per month or maybe only one or two a year. Headaches may be continuous and last for days or weeks and may or may not fluctuate in intensity.

For some, lying down in a dark, quiet room is a must. For others, life can continue on like normal. Headaches are a major reason for missed work or school days as well as for doctor visits. The "cost" of headaches is enormous—running into the billions of dollars per year in the United States (US) in both direct costs and productivity losses. Indirect costs such as the potential future costs in children with headaches who miss school and the associated interference with their academic progress are much more difficult to calculate.

There are MANY types of headaches, which are classified into types. With each type, there is a different cause or group of causes. For example, migraine headaches, which affect about 12% of the US population (both children and adults), are vascular in nature—where the blood vessels dilate or enlarge and irritate nerve-sensitive tissues inside the head. This usually results in throbbing, pulsating pain often on one side of the head and can include nausea and/or vomiting. Some migraine sufferers have an "aura" such as a flashing or bright light that occurs within 10-15 minutes prior to the onset while other migraine sufferers do not have an aura.

The tension-type headache is the most common type and as the name implies, is triggered by stress or some type of tension. The intensity ranges between mild and severe, usually on both sides of the head and often begin during adolescence and peak around age 30, affecting women slightly more than men. These can be episodic (come and go, ten to fifteen times a month, lasting 30 min. to several days) or chronic (more than fifteen times a month over a three-month period).

Are Headaches and Dizziness a "Dangerous Combination"?

Last month, we discussed some startling new research that found that lightheadedness upon standing up (orthostatic hypotension) may be more serious than previously thought. This month, we'll look specifically at headache AND dizziness and if we should we be concerned about this combination of complaints and if so, when?

A team of researchers from Johns Hopkins University reviewed past medical records of 187,188 patients presenting to over 1,000 emergency departments (EDs) between 2008 and 2009. They found the combination of headache and dizziness—especially in women, minorities, and young patients—was a potential signal of an impending stroke!

Specifically, they reported that 12.7% of people complaining of headache and dizziness were later admitted for stroke and had been misdiagnosed and inappropriately sent home from the ED within the previous 30 days. Patients were told they had a "benign condition" such as inner ear infection or migraine, and in some cases, they weren't given a diagnosis at all. Slightly less than half of this population had a stroke within seven days and over half had a stoke within the first 48 hours of the initial pre-stroke ED presentation!

The study reported that women were 33% and minorities 20-30% more likely to be misdiagnosed, suggesting gender and racial disparities may play a role. The researchers estimate that doctors miss 15,000 to 165,000 strokes that result in harm to the patient each year.

Studies have found that the early diagnosis and quick treatment of strokes is critical in reducing serious residuals in patients having a transient ischemic attach (TIA), sometimes referred to as a "mini-stroke" or "pre-stroke." TIAs are often pre-cursors to a more catastrophic stroke leading to death or permanent disability without appropriate treatment.

Again, to put this in perspective, MANY people present to healthcare providers with headaches and dizziness with NO relationship to stroke—about 87%—though it is sometimes not

60

possible to know whether a potentially dangerous problem may arise in the near future. The good news is that it usually does not!

The importance of this study is to alert both healthcare providers AND patients of the potential risk. When in doubt, it's ALWAYS best to seek out multiple opinions. An MRI may be the best way to confirm the most common type of stroke (according the study reviewed above), as a CT scan may not show the brain changes early on and could lead to false reassurance.

Tension vs. Migraine: What's the Difference?

Most likely, everyone reading this article has had a headache at one time or another. The American Headache Society reports that nearly 40% of the population suffers from episodic headaches each year while 3% have chronic tension-type headaches. The United States Department of Health and·Human Services estimates that 29.5 million Americans experience migraines, but tension headaches are more common than migraines at a frequency of 5 to 1. Knowing the difference between the two is important, as the proper diagnosis can guide treatment in the right direction.

TENSION HEADACHES: These typically result in a steady ache and tightness located in the neck, particularly at the base of the skull, which can irritate the upper cervical nerve roots resulting in radiating pain and/or numbness into the head. At times, the pain can reach the eyes but often stops at the top of the head. Common triggers include stress, muscle strain, or anxiety.

MIGRAINE HEADACHES: Migraines are often much more intense, severe, and sometimes incapacitating. They usually remain on one side of the head and are associated with nausea and/or vomiting. An "aura", or a pre-headache warning, often comes with symptoms such as a bright flashing light, ringing or noise in the ears, a visual floater, and more. For migraine headaches, there is often a strong family history, which indicates genetics may play a role in their origin.

There are many causes for headaches. Commonly, they include lack of sleep and/or stress and they can also result from a recent injury—such as a car accident, and/or a sports injury—especially when accompanied by a concussion.

Certain things can "trigger" a migraine including caffeine, chocolate, citrus fruits, cured meats, dehydration, depression, diet (skipping meals), dried fish, dried fruit, exercise (excessive), eyestrain, fatigue (extreme), food additives (nitrites, nitrates, MSG), lights (bright, flickering, glare), menstruation, some medications, noise, nuts, odors, onions, altered sleep, stress, watching TV, red wine/alcohol, weather, etc.

Posture is also a very important consideration. A forward head carriage is not only related to headaches, but also neck and back pain. We've previously pointed out that every inch (2.54 cm) the average 12 pound head (5.44 kg) shifts forwards adds an EXTRA ten pounds (4.5 kg) of load on the neck and upper back muscles to keep the head upright.

So, what can be done for people who suffer from headaches? First, research shows chiropractic care is highly effective for patients with both types of headaches. Spinal manipulation, deep tissue release techniques, and nutritional counseling are common approaches utilized by chiropractors. Patients are also advised to use some of these self-management strategies at home as part of their treatment plan: the use of ice, self-trigger point therapy, exercise (especially strengthening the deep neck flexors), and nutritional supplements.

Headaches, Hygiene and Pillows

We hear about dental hygiene and how to eat right, but when was the last time you considered if you slept well in a way that does not stress the spine. Most of us know it's important to avoid head and neck trauma because serious and devastating injuries can occur. Less understood, are how minor and cumulative stresses over time can affect the soft tissues in the neck.

If you have never suffered a neck trauma, then maintaining good neck habits is less critical. But most of us have had a few kinks in the neck over the years, and we tend to suffer when problems are not prevented in the first place.

Keeping the neck supple and flexible with daily stretches can help many patients. Others may need to do daily controlled exercises to keep the muscles strong. A doctor can advise you on your specific needs. It's important to be diagnosed properly before starting any stretching or exercising program.

Ever wonder why your neck might be stiff in the morning? Maintaining good spinal hygiene while sleeping is also important. Eight hours of bad posture can be a significant problem.

Because there is naturally an arch formed in the neck when you lay on your back, a pillow can be designed to support the middle of your neck. These types of pillows are called cervical pillows or neck support pillows. Researchers from Canada (J Can Chiro Assoc, 2004) used a semi-custom pillow in patients with neck pain (with or without headache) to test its effectiveness. The patients used the pillows over four weeks. In this randomized and controlled study, the patients who used the pillows had significantly less pain in the morning. They also looked at the patients' ability/disability over time and discovered that this also improved in the group that used the custom pillows.

Our clinic provides patients with spinal hygiene exercises and advice to care for problems over time. This can be key to you avoiding re-aggravation of your condition and to prevent problems from occurring in the first place. Many headache patients seem to benefit when they pay attention to the stresses on their neck. It can be looking at a computer screen with the head down or something as simple as the type of pillow you use while sleeping.

Headaches: Causes and Promising Solutions

Chronic headaches are a mystery to most of us. Why they occur seems to be the most common question. Some patients' headaches can be easily explained, but many seem to get headaches for no apparent reason. An often overlooked cause of headaches is the spine and spinal trauma. How does this occur?

Delicate connective tissue link the muscles in your neck area around your spinal cord. One theory is that tensions can develop in these structures producing head pain. Another possibility to consider is that of forward head posture.

Forward head posture is present when the head is thrust forward in the classic bad posture pose (a little like a turtle neck), taking out the natural curve in the neck. Since the head is quite heavy (10-14 lbs), the muscles in the back of the neck have to counter this weight. When the neck muscles resist the load of the head, they can develop tensions, knots (trigger points), and sometimes spasms.

Another cause for headaches is a joint injury/sprain that can occur after whiplash trauma. Over time, this may lead to joint blockage where there is not the normal free and fluid motion from side to side. In many cases, other joints must compensate for this lack of movement with hypermobility. In reaction, your muscles can become tense in these areas to protect the spine from unnatural movements.

Since these types of disorders are so common in society, they should be ruled out before leaning towards long-term pharmaceutical treatments. It is always important to have an accurate diagnosis before proceeding with treatment. If your headaches have become chronic and just never seem to go away, it is a sign that you are not getting at the cause of the problem.

Correcting neck disorders when they occur is always the best choice. But when a headache seems to come out of nowhere and there is a history of neck trauma in your past, treating the neck can and should be a part of your headache management strategy. At the minimum, the neck needs to be examined.

Chiropractic care has been shown in multiple clinical trials to help patients with both tension-type and migraine headaches. In these studies, the neck or cervical spine is adjusted based on local problems of poor posture and mobility.

Headaches From Forward Head Posture

John Q. Public has been trained to believe that a headache is a problem in the head and relief comes in a bottle.

While it's true that pain medications can bring relief for a pounding headache, they rarely get at the actual cause of the problem. You have to also consider the long-term problems that can occur when you take these types of pills for years or even decades. Some long-term complications include stomach bleeding, liver and kidney problems. Plus there is the problem of not actually correcting anything and instead masking the symptoms. Pain pills are not one of the five food groups.

For many patients, the problem is not one in the head, but may have a spinal cause. Let me explain how this works…. Normally, the neck is balanced over the shoulders in an upright manner. Some people, however, develop forward head posture where the head protrudes out away from the shoulder girdle-it looks like the bad posture your mother told to avoid. This type of posture is often seen in computer operators and others who bend over to do their work. Whiplash injuries can also create this forward head posture by disrupting the natural curve of the neck.

Over time the muscles at the back of the neck become tight and start to tug and pull at the base of the skull. This can cause head pain. Sometimes it's a dull ache with a burning type of pain full of tension. In other patients, the headache may be more throbbing and to one side. The important thing is to address the actual cause of the problem. This is where chiropractic care is key. By correcting the forward head posture, the head is more balanced over the shoulders. Many patients will report less tension in their shoulder and upper back muscles which were really working over time.

Is It All In My Head?

Probably not is what most research indicates. Most head pains are caused by problems outside the head: too little sleep, too much alcohol, or too much stress. Rarely is there a trauma in the head or a stroke causing the pain. More common, neck injuries from whiplash or sporting accidents can cause headaches. This is because the spinal joints have been sprained and the nerves are irritated. There may also be some stretch to the tough linings around the spinal cord.

Many headache sufferers understand that neck pain and tension often come with the head pain. For them, the idea of neck problems linked to headaches is understandable. When you can understand that the location of the pain (in your head) is not necessarily where the problem is located, you've taken a big step in understanding how the body works. Because mechanical neck and back problems can cause areas distant to show pain, it is easy to get lead astray down the endless path of pills and potions.

A scoliosis in the lower spine will need to be compensated for above and this often has to occur in the neck. Taken a step further, when a problem affects the pelvis or hip, such as a short leg, the eyes will try to level to correct for the tilt below. This is why sometimes adjustments to the neck region alone will not fix a difficult headache case.

If there are biomechanical problems below the neck this can affect the overall effectiveness of the care. For these reasons the chiropractor needs to address the full spine when seeking a cause for a patient's headache.

It is important to look at the scientific evidence behind a treatment if you're making important health care decisions. You need to weigh both the pros and cons of anything, and you also want to get at the root cause of any problem.

In migraine and tension headaches, the evidence shows that chiropractic care will decrease the pain as quickly as powerful medications, but without the side effects associated with drugs that only cover up the symptoms. Although more research is definitely needed, for those who want a holistic and natural approach, chiropractic care is the clear choice.

"My Head Feels Heavy at the End of the Day –What Can I Do?"

The head is a large and heavy part of a person. In a child, the head can account for ¼ of their height. In the adult, the head weighs 10-14 pounds, and this load has to be balanced by the strength of the neck muscles. In normal upright posture, there is a forward curve to the neck, and this curve provides the perfect balance between strength and mobility. Unfortunately, this curve can be disrupted by whiplash and other traumas that damage the delicate ligaments and disks. This results in a straight or "military" neck.

When a person bends their head forward to read or type, the neck begins to straighten and the weight of the head must be countered by the pull of the muscles at the back of the neck. If the person does this all day, because they work at a computer for example, then the muscles never get a break. Knots, tightness or spasm of the muscles will increase and cause a neck ache. The person may feel a tightness or pain around the head because the muscles pull at the base of the skull. These are the symptoms of what is called a tension-type headache.

Usually the shoulder muscles are also involved and tight. Over time this forward head posture can become more permanent and a "round back" may also develop. More than just bad appearance, poor posture causes the spinal cord and nerves to become stretched resulting in pain. Poor posture may also cause the spine to prematurely deteriorate, called degeneration, which results in thin disks.

Forward head posture and bad neck curves can be diagnosed by x-ray and by observing the patient from the side. If forward head posture is detected, it usually means there is some stretch to the ligaments.

The answer cannot be found in a bottle of pain pills. Although they can block pain, the consequences are quite severe. First, they mask the cause of the symptoms and lead the patient away from the actual cause of the head pain. In addition, pain pills can cause stomach bleeding and kidney damage when taken for long periods of time.

There are other causes for tension-type headaches and the 'heavy' feeling of the head. Certain rare diseases and high blood pressure can also make the head hurt. This is why it is important to have the cause of your problem properly diagnosed. Chiropractic doctors have extensively studied both spinal problems that cause headaches, as well as the more rare diseases, which occasionally cause the same symptoms.

"I Keep Taking Ibuprofen and Acetaminophen and My Migraines Are Getting Worse, Not Better"

It is difficult to not know someone who suffers from chronic headaches or migraines. In 2004, the percentage of adults who experienced a severe headache or migraine during the preceding 3 months was 18%. Migraine headaches, which are characterized by painful, disabling, and recurring symptoms, have no known proven cause, treatment, or cure. They occur more often in women than men and in one ten year period, the proportion of adults with migraine increased 64-77%.

Chronic migraine headaches are classified either as ``common'' or ``classical.'' Symptoms of the common migraine headache include nausea, dizziness, fever, and general malaise. The classical migraine headache is most noted for an aura that immediately precedes the headache. This aura could be visual or auditory. In addition, the classical migraine headache is characterized by a relatively short duration (less than or equal to 12 hours) compared with the common migraine headache (up to 4 days).

Although clinical studies have not clearly defined the cause of chronic migraine headaches, potential risk factors include: diet, allergy, air quality, and stress. Many patients use complementary treatments such as chiropractic care. Recent studies have shown that patients who have had neck trauma such as whiplash are at greater risk for headache. Cervicogenic headache is a term for when the neck or cervical spine causes pain to be experienced in the head. Usually the neck or upper back region has muscle tightness and limited mobility.

In tension-type headaches there is a great deal of muscle

tension in the neck, and the headache begins as a band of tension around the head, rather than a severe pulsating pain on one side as seen in migraine.

Whatever the type of headache, most patients have suffered for years and have been taking many pain pills such as ibuprofen and aspirin with few results. Recent research has shown that when these medications are consumed for long periods, they can actually cause a rebound effect and increase headache frequency. The headache can initially get worse as the patient has the medication withdrawn. In addition to actually increasing the severity of the headache, long-term use of these medications can cause organ damage to the stomach, liver, or kidney.

It is important to remember that a headache is a symptom that tells you something is wrong. Covering up the symptom will not solve the problem. Physical approaches involving spine posture are important to consider and are generally preferred to injections, sprays, and medications. A seeming endless diet of pain medications with unknown safety is not the answer for patients with headache.

Headaches: Causes and Promising Solutions

Chronic headaches are a mystery to most of us. Why they occur seems to be the most common question. Some patients' headaches can be easily explained, but many seem to get headaches for no apparent reason. An often overlooked cause of headaches is the spine and spinal trauma. How does this occur?

Delicate connective tissue link the muscles in your neck area around your spinal cord. One theory is that tensions can develop in these structures producing head pain. Another possibility to consider is that of forward head posture.

Forward head posture is present when the head is thrust forward in the classic bad posture pose (a little like a turtle neck), taking out the natural curve in the neck. Since the head is quite heavy (10-14 lbs), the muscles in the back of the neck have to counter this weight. When the neck muscles resist the load of the head, they can develop tensions, knots (trigger points), and sometimes spasms.

Another cause for headaches is a joint injury/sprain that can occur after whiplash trauma. Over time, this may lead to joint blockage where there is not the normal free and fluid motion from side to side. In many cases, other joints must compensate for this lack of movement with hypermobility. In reaction, your muscles can become tense in these areas to protect the spine from unnatural movements.

Since these types of disorders are so common in society, they should be ruled out before leaning towards long-term pharmaceutical treatments. It is always important to have an accurate diagnosis before proceeding with treatment. If your headaches have become chronic and just never seem to go away, it is a sign that you are not getting at the cause of the problem.

Correcting neck disorders when they occur is always the best choice. But when a headache seems to come out of nowhere and there is a history of neck trauma in your past, treating the neck can and should be a part of your headache management strategy. At the minimum, the neck needs to be examined.

Chiropractic care has been shown in multiple clinical trials to help patients with both tension-type and migraine headaches. In these studies, the neck or cervical spine is adjusted based on local problems of poor posture and mobility.

CARPAL TUNNEL SYNDROME (CTS)

Carpal Tunnel Syndrome – Let's Get the FACTS! (Part 1)

If tingling/numbness primarily affects your thumb, index, third, and ring fingers, it very well could be carpal tunnel syndrome, or CTS. Chances are you've probably had this condition for months or even longer but it's been more of a nuisance than a "major problem" and therefore, you probably haven't "bothered" having it checked out. Let's take a look at some "facts" about CTS!

WHAT IS CTS? CTS is basically a pinched nerve (the median nerve) that occurs on the palm side of the wrist that innervates the three middle fingers and the thumb on the palm side. This nerve starts in the neck, runs through the shoulder to enter the arm, and travels down the palm side forearm through the carpal tunnel. The carpal tunnel is made up by eight small bones (called "carpal bones") that form the roof and walls of the tunnel. The floor of the tunnel is a ligament called the transverse carpal ligament. The median nerve lies immediately on the floor, and deeper inside the tunnel are nine tendons that connect the muscles of our forearm to the fingers, which allow us to make a fist and grip. When swelling occurs inside the tunnel, the nerve is pinched against the floor (ligament) and symptoms occur.

SYMPTOMS OF CTS: Symptoms typically start gradually with tingling, numbness, burning, itching, or a "half-sleep" feeling in the palm of the hand, thumb, and middle three fingers. The fingers can feel swollen and weak, though "swelling" is usually NOT visible. CTS can occur in one or both hands, but it is usually worse in the dominant hand. Initially, you may only notice symptoms at night or in the morning. As CTS worsens, sleep interruptions, grip weakness, difficulty distinguishing hot from cold, increased pain, pain radiating up the arm, and more may occur.

CAUSES OF CTS: There are many causes of CTS that often occur in combination: 1) Heredity or genetics — being born with a smaller wrist than others; 2) Trauma — a fall on the arm/hand (sprain or fracture); 3) Overuse of the arms/hands (like repetitive line work, serving tables, or using a computer), 4) Hormonal causes — during menstruation, with pregnancy, during menopause, diabetes, hypothyroid, overactive pituitary gland; 5) Rheumatoid arthritis; 6) Fluid retention; 7) Cysts, tumors, or spurs inside the tunnel; 8) Vibrating tools, 9) Hobbies such as knitting, sewing, crocheting; 10) sports; or 11) an "Insidious" or unknown cause!

CTS RISK FACTORS: 1) Gender: Women are three times more likely to develop CTS, possibly because they generally have a smaller carpal tunnel than men, in addition to hormonal differences; 2) Diabetes or other metabolic disorders; 3) Adults, especially >50 years old; 4) Job demands.

CTS DIAGNOSIS: Your doctor of chiropractic will review your patient history and then evaluate the neck, shoulder, arm, and hand, as ALL can be involved in producing CTS-like symptoms. He/she may also order blood tests (to check for diabetes, thyroid levels, rheumatoid arthritis, etc.) and/or an EMG/NCV (electromyogram/nerve conduction studies) to test for nerve damage.

Carpal Tunnel Syndrome vs. Cubital Tunnel Syndrome

Carpal Tunnel Syndrome (CTS) belongs to a group of disorders referred to as "cumulative trauma disorders," or CTDs. The word "cumulative" refers to the cause being repetitive motion, usually fast and prolonged. Over time, the wear and tear on the upper extremities accumulates and symptoms begin to occur and possibly worsen. This can result in changes in movement intended to avoid further injury that then overstress another part of the arm, which can lead to a second injury. Like dominos, injury after injury can eventually result in multiple conditions between the neck and hand. Let's take a look at two of the more common CTDs...

Carpal Tunnel Syndrome (CTS) is the most well known of the CTDs because the thumb, index, third, and fourth ring finger comprise 90% of the hand's function. This part of the hand is innervated by the median nerve that travels through the carpal tunnel at the wrist. When injured, it can make fine motor movements, like tying your shoe, difficult-to-impossible! Our grip strength is also greatly affected by a pinch of the median nerve, so dropping coffee cups, difficulty removing a gallon milk jug from the refrigerator, and the ability to lift and carry are all compromised. Some risk factors for CTS include: 1) Age over 50; 2) Female gender; 3) Obesity; 4) Working in a highly repetitive motion type of job (assembly line work, meat/poultry plants, typing); 5) The presence of other CTDs such as forearm, wrist, or hand tendonitis; and 6) Metabolic conditions such as thyroid disease (hypothyroidism), diabetes, rheumatoid arthritis, and more. Management strategies include: 1) Night use of a wrist splint (i.e., rest); 2) chiropractic manipulation of the small joints of the wrist and hand, and often, the elbow, shoulder, and neck; 3) Muscle and tendon myofascial release / mobilization techniques; 4) Management of any underlying metabolic condition (like hypothyroid disease and diabetes); and 5) Anti-inflammatory measures (ginger, turmeric, boswellia, bioflavinoids, vitamin B6, ice massage over the palm side of the wrist). NOTE: Recent studies have reported the use of NSAIDs—non-steroidal anti-inflammatory drugs like Advil (ibuprofen), Aleve (Naproxen), and aspirin—can interfere with and prolong the healing process. Chiropractic care may also include the use of modalities such as low level laser therapy, pulsed magnetic field, ultrasound, and/or electrical stimulation. Your doctor may order an EMG/NCV (electromyogram/nerve conduction velocity) if the case is not responding appropriately.

Surgical intervention is the LAST RESORT but frequently, conservative chiropractic care yields satisfying results!

Cubital Tunnel Syndrome (Ulnar Nerve Entrapment – UNE): This is similar to CTS but it involves the ulnar nerve being pinched at the inner elbow (near where the "funny" bone is located). The big difference here is that the numbness/tingling involves the pinky side of the fourth and fifth fingers (NOT the thumb, index, third, or thumb-side of the fourth finger). Remember, you can have BOTH CTS and ulnar nerve entrapment (UNE) at the same time, in which case all five fingers may be involved. Causes are similar as CTS, but a more recently identified cause is called "cell phone elbow" due to the prolonged elbow flexed/bent position while using a phone. An overnight splint keeping the elbow straight as well as a wrist splint can be very effective. Otherwise, the treatment is similar to that described for CTS and it is frequently easily managed with non-surgical chiropractic care!

What Exercises Can I do for CTS?

Carpal Tunnel Syndrome (CTS) is the leading cause of numbness to the middle three fingers and thumb and affects millions of Americans each year. There are MANY potential causes of CTS, and these causes can be unclear or multi-factorial. We have discussed the importance of night splints and what chiropractic can do for CTS in the recent past. This month, let's look at what YOU can do for CTS.

"Self-help" concepts are VERY important as they empower YOU to gain control of your condition's signs and symptoms, thus placing less reliance on those of us who manage (in this case) CTS. There is a time for "PRICE" or, Protect, Rest, Ice, Compress, Elevate, such as when most activities make symptoms worse. This is the time for splinting, reducing activities of daily living (which sometimes includes work restrictions), and the use of ice cupping or massage. Patients should initiate movement or exercise-based approaches as soon as such activities can be tolerated. Here are four different exercises you can do:

1. Fist / "Bear Claw" / Open Wide Hand: This is a three-step exercise, and you can start or stop on any of the three "steps." A. FIST: Make a fist and squeeze as tightly as tolerated; B. BEAR CLAW: Starting from the fist position (A), open only the palm of the hand (keep your thumb and fingers bent but straighten the big knuckle joints at the base of the fingers); C. OPEN WIDE: Straighten and spread ALL your finger joints by opening up your hand as much as possible and feel for a good stretch in the palm. HOLD each position for one to five seconds (vary the "speed" of moving between the three positions – fast, medium, and slow; emphasize what feels best if you have a preference). Repeat five to ten times or until your hands feel looser.

2. "Church Steeple": Place your hands together in front of you ("prayer position") touching the pads of the thumbs and all four fingertips together and spread your fingers as wide as possible. Next, separate your palms as far as you can while applying pressure against your finger/thumb tips and repeat. Alter the speed and number of repetitions until your hands feel stretched out.

3. "Shake and Flick": Simply shake your hands as if you just washed them and you're shaking the water off to "air dry" them. Again, alter the speed and reps until they feel loosened up.

4. Forearm Stretches: Place one arm out in front, elbow straight, and fingers pointed straight, palm up (first set). Reach with the opposite hand and pull the fingers, hand, and wrist down and back towards you until you feel a strong "pull" in your forearm muscles. Hold until the forearm muscles feels stretched (5-10 seconds). Repeat this with the palm facing down for the second set to stretch the opposite (extensor) forearm muscles.

Do these on each side two to three times each (even the "good" side) EVERY HOUR (or as often as possible). Think about what you do on a daily basis and if you work in a repetitive manner (on the job or a hobby at home), try to do these exercises DURING THE REPETITIVE ACTIVITY to help keep your symptoms from getting out of control. If you can alter the position or speed of a work or avocational activity, do so for long-term prevention purposes!

If you cannot gain control of your CTS condition, you may need additional treatment options of which chiropractic offers a safe, non-surgical approach.

Non-Surgical Treatment Approaches for CTS

Non-surgical treatment approaches for carpal tunnel syndrome (CTS) aim to remove pressure on the median nerve where it's pinched. In a recent review of the literature published on "passive modalities" (non-surgical treatment approaches) for CTS, researchers reviewed studies published between 1990 and 2015 for information on which non-surgical treatment approaches work best. Topping the list is the use of various types of night splints – wrist braces worn at night to prevent bending of the wrist during sleep. The evidence found that night splints were less effective than surgery in the short-term (up to six months) but more effective over the long-term (at 12 and 18 months)!

They did not find studies with a "low risk of bias" (no randomized controlled trial-types of studies) regarding other passive modalities such as ultrasound and electrical stim and hence, they conclude that better quality studies must be conducted before conclusions can be made regarding most of the passive modalities frequently utilized in the management of CTS.

A 2010 study found mobilization treatments and exercises (tendon gliding & nerve gliding) were helpful WHEN patients complied with the treatments and the recommended exercises. Manual therapies, or "hands-on" treatments, are a feature of chiropractic care. Chiropractic treatment for patients with CTS also includes night bracing in addition to manipulation, mobilization, exercise training, nutrition, and ergonomic / workstation modifications, and whole body health awareness.

Doctors of chiropractic understand these non-surgical approaches have limitations. This is why they work with allied healthcare providers when pharmaceutical and/or surgical intervention is appropriate. They may also frequently consult with neurologists for tests such as EMG/NCV (an electrical test that measures the degree of nerve damage) to better understand the patient's condition. In short, chiropractic offers a multi-modal approach of care, and chiropractors will work with others in the patient's best interest.

When Should I Consider Surgery for CTS?

Carpal Tunnel Syndrome (CTS) affects 3% of the adults in the United States and is the most common of the "entrapment neuropathies" (pinched nerves in the arms or legs). Treatment for CTS is frequently delayed because the symptoms are usually mild at first and progress gradually. Because CTS symptoms may be more advanced by the time a patient seeks treatment, he or she may think surgery is the only viable option. So, when should a patient consider surgery for CTS?

CTS has many causes. Hence, managing it relies on an accurate diagnosis. The condition is associated with the following: female (4x more likely than male), obesity, rheumatoid arthritis, pregnancy, diabetes, thyroid dysfunction, renal dialysis (amyloid), and trauma, especially fractures. Certain medications such as oral contraceptives and other hormone replacement therapies can also increase the risk of developing CTS. In cases with a strong family history of CTS, a hereditary risk factor may also exist. Because compression of the median nerve at locations other than the wrist can also lead to carpal tunnel-like symptoms, it's important for a doctor to check the course of the median nerve from its origin in the neck down to the wrist.

So WHEN should a non-surgical approach be used? Short answer: almost always. Exceptions include acute carpal tunnel syndrome, which occurs rarely but should be considered urgent since permanent problems may QUICKLY result if it's NOT surgically managed. One example is when a wrist fracture places compression on the median nerve. Bleeding (from any cause) into the carpal tunnel is another scenario when emergency surgery is necessary. A third (rare but serious) situation is if infection is present in the carpal tunnel. More commonly, the decision to have vs. not have surgery depends on the amount of nerve damage (weakness, pain, numbness/tingling), the resulting loss of function or inability to perform desired work or home activities, and the length of time CTS has been a problem. The AAOS (American Academy of Orthopaedic Surgeons) recommends a course of nonsurgical treatment (as do most guidelines) with treatment options that include the use of bracing (wrist cock-up splint), local steroid injection, or ultrasound. When other conditions co-occur with carpal tunnel syndrome symptoms, the AAOS found insufficient research evidence to provide specific recommendations. This means a patient should WAIT on surgery until the co-existing condition/s (like diabetes, double crush, hormone imbalance, and/or work place/ergonomic problems) are properly managed to see if their symptoms persist.

With this in mind, consider a four-to-six week trial (or longer if you are responding and satisfied) of non-surgical care prior to consulting with a surgeon. A 2010 study described conservative treatment options to include physical therapy, bracing, steroid injection, and alternative medicine (like chiropractic). More research is needed to make strong recommendations for treatments such as exercise, yoga, acupuncture, and lasers. The authors of the study do cite mobilization exercises (tendon gliding & nerve gliding) as being helpful WHEN patients comply with the treatments and the recommended exercises (a definite problem). Chiropractic management includes bracing, manipulation, mobilization, exercise training, nutrition, and ergonomic / work station modifications. Doctors of chiropractic understand the limitations to these approaches and work with other healthcare providers when pharmaceutical and/or surgical intervention may be needed.

Why Should I Exercise For Carpal Tunnel Syndrome?

Carpal Tunnel Syndrome (CTS) is an EXTREMELY common condition that can affect anyone at any age. In fact, there's a strong probability that up to 50% of the people reading this today have or have had symptoms of CTS at some point in time and 10% or more have been treated for it! We have recently discussed various non-surgical treatment approaches for managing CTS but the question of WHY exercises should be included in that program remains a mystery to many!

In review of the anatomy of the carpal tunnel, we've got nine tendons that are the "shoe strings" that connect the muscles in the palm-side forearm to the fingers traveling through the tunnel along with the infamous MEDIAN NERVE—the culprit creating the numbness and tingling associated with CTS. The bony "roof" of the tunnel is made up of eight carpal bones that connect our forearm to our hand and allow us to bend the wrist in many directions. Without these eight little bones, we would not be able to bend our wrist at all! The "floor" of the tunnel is the transverse carpal ligament, and the median nerve lies directly on top of it. CTS occurs when the contents within the tunnel swell and apply pressure that pushes the median nerve into the floor, which is common when the wrist is bent, such as when sleeping with our hand curled under our chin at night – hence the reason for a night splint (cock-up brace) to prevent nighttime bending.

Now that we have a picture of the tunnel in our mind, exercises for CTS will make more sense. CTS occurs when forceful, repetitive tasks are performed over a lengthy period of time (examples include practicing a musical instrument, assembly line work, carpentry, etc.). The FRICTION between the tendons ("shoe strings") inside the tunnel creates swelling and that results in tightness.

EXERCISE #1 is ICING using an ice cube or frozen Dixie cup of water and rubbing it over the tunnel. First you will feel COLD, then BURNING, then ACHING, and finally NUMBNESS ("C-BAN"). Quit at numbness as the next stage of cooling is frostbite! Many of you may not look at "ice massage" as an exercise, but it's very important!

EXERCISE #2 – Stand near a countertop, place the palm-side of your fingers on the edge of the counter and push until your wrist is bent backwards as far as you can stand it while keeping your elbow straight. Now reach across with your other hand and pull your thumb backwards as far as possible. Can you feel the "pull" in your mid forearm up to the elbows? GOOD! Hold that for three to five seconds, rest for five seconds and repeat it three times. Do this on both sides, even if the other hand is "normal" so you can feel the difference between the "tight" CTS side vs. the normal arm. CTS is often bilateral so you may not notice a difference. Now, set the timer on your smartphone to ring every hour to remind you to do this throughout the work day.

EXERCISE #3 is the fist / "bear claw" / hand open sequence. First, make a tight fist, followed by opening your hand while keeping the fingers flexed/bent, followed by opening the hand and fingers fully. Hold each position for two to three seconds and go through the sequence as often as needed (usually two to three times a session, multiple times a day) and do BOTH sides at the same time.

Why do these help? They break up adhesions between the tendons, their sheaths, and the surrounding tissues, and these exercises also force you to take "mini-breaks" during a busy day, which can reduce swelling in the carpal tunnel.

Facts About Carpal Tunnel Syndrome and Sleep

Have you ever woken up at night with numbness and tingling in your fingers and had to climb out of bed and shake your hands, flick your fingers, and/or rub your arms to "…wake them up?" Well, you're not alone! In fact, this is one of the more common and often one of the FIRST symptoms of Carpal Tunnel Syndrome (CTS). So, WHY does this happen?

The "carpal tunnel" is literally just a tunnel that MANY components of the body travel through on the way to the hand. The walls are made from eight small "carpal" bones and the "floor" of the tunnel is made by the transverse carpal ligament. These structures vary in size and shape and differ between males and females, which may be one reason CTS is more common among women than men. The contents of the tunnel include eight tendons that connect the muscles in the forearm to the index, third, ring, and pinky fingers. A ninth tendon that connects to the muscle that flexes the thumb also travels through the tunnel along with blood vessels. Perhaps most importantly, the median nerve that supplies sensation and strength to the palm side fingers (index, third and ring fingers) and the palm of the hand also travels through the carpal tunnel. The tendons to the fingers and thumb are "sheathed" and can swell due to the friction created by the tendon rapidly moving in the tight sheath. This is one reason why people who work in an occupation that requires fast, repetitive hand movements (such as assembly line work, carpentry, food preparation, for example) will often have problems with carpal tunnel syndrome.

The pressure inside the wrist normally doubles when it is fully bent either forwards or backwards. However, because there is already greater pressure in the affected carpal tunnel of individuals with CTS (due to swollen tendons, for example), the pressure inside the carpal tunnel can increase much more when the wrist is bent. This added pressure can exacerbate the symptoms normally associated with CTS—including numbness and tingling in the hands and fingers—especially when the wrist is bent for a prolonged period of time, such as during sleep.

Treatment associated with carpal tunnel syndrome includes the use of a night wrist cock-up splint, which keeps the wrist from flexing or extending during sleep and helps the swelling inside the carpal tunnel abate. Cock-up splints are not typically worn during the day, as they tend to interfere too much with normal activity and may actually worsen the condition depending on the length of time and the type of work the person is performing. Driving will often increase symptoms, and use of the cock-up splint can be effective during this time.

Chiropractic management offers a unique form of treatment called manipulation and mobilization that is applied to the fingers, hand, wrist, forearm, and any other area where nerve compression might be present, which frequently includes the cervical spine/neck region. The shoulder and elbow may also require care.

Anti-inflammatory measures including ice massage over the wrist and anti-inflammatory herbal preparations such as ginger, turmeric, and/or digestive enzymes taken between meals can help. Modifying the ergonomics of a CTS patient's workstation is a good idea in order to reduce the repetitive strain commonly associated with chronic carpal tunnel syndrome.

Carpal Tunnel Syndrome and Neck Pain

The Great Mystery!

Carpal Tunnel Syndrome (CTS) develops when the median nerve is pinched at the palm-side of the wrist causing numbness in the index, third, and thumb-side half of the ring/fourth finger. Since the median nerve passes through the neck, it's possible that dysfunction in the neck can interfere with the median nerve, resulting in carpal tunnel syndrome-like symptoms. Sometimes the median nerve can be "pinched" in both the neck and the wrist in what's known as double crush syndrome.

Though many patients benefit from both surgical and non-surgical CTS treatment approaches, it is not uncommon for the results to fall short of a total resolution of symptoms. In these unsuccessful cases, it's possible the median nerve is "pinched" at one or more locations other than the area the treatment focused on. In some cases, the hand symptoms and other signs of CTS can improve following treatment to relieve cervical dysfunction. The opposite can also be true with neck pain and related symptoms improving when the carpal tunnel is treated.

The concept of "differential diagnosis" has to do with considering multiple possible causes that can create similar symptoms, and one by one, ruling "in" or "out" each diagnosis by performing various tests with the ultimate goal of coming away with one solid diagnosis. Of course, the problem with this is that there is often more than one diagnosis at play, and in such cases we must determine which one is primary vs. secondary.

Taking our topic this month as an example, a chiropractor may often see cervical spine x-ray findings such as degenerative disk spaces, osteoarthritic spurring, or narrowing of the foramen that the spinal nerves pass through in route to the arm and hand. However, they may not be sure if these findings are "clinically important" or even contribute to a "cervical radiculopathy" or pinched nerve in the neck. It's possible to see these same x-ray findings in patients with no radiating arm symptoms whatsoever.

Similarly, patients with radiating arm / hand complaints may have NONE of these findings! The same holds true with bulging and/or herniated disks in the neck because these may or may NOT cause any radiating symptoms. When a chiropractor is able to reproduce arm and hand symptoms during an examination of the neck that are similar to CTS, this increases the doctor's suspicion that at least a portion of the hand complaints may be attributed to nerve compression from the neck. When both neck and wrist findings co-exist, tests like EMG (electromyography) and NCV (nerve conduction velocity) can really help in some cases, but in other instances, the degree of nerve loss (the amount of damage) may not be enough to be accurately assessed with such diagnostic tools.

The "bottom line" is that all health care practitioners start "conservative" and wait until all approaches have been exhausted prior to recommending surgery. As described in previous articles, there are MANY non-surgical approaches that chiropractors can provide and you owe it to yourself to try these conservative approaches first!

Carpal Tunnel Syndrome –

WHAT YOU NEED TO KNOW!

Carpal Tunnel Syndrome (CTS) develops from a nerve problem in the wrist (the median nerve) and is NOT a "muscle problem" like some people believe. That is not to say the median nerve cannot be trapped and pinched by muscles. When this occurs, the condition is labeled with a different name, depending on which muscle(s) are pinching the nerve or where the entrapment is located. Here are some more FACTS about CTS that you need to know:

SYMPTOMS: CTS complaints include numbness, pain, tingling, and/or weakness of the hand (especially fingers two, three, and four), and while this can be constant, it usually comes and goes.

ONSET: CTS usually comes on gradually. However, the length of time over which it progresses can be HIGHLY VARIABLE. It can take weeks, months, or even years before the patient consults with their chiropractor or family doctor.

CAUSE: There are MANY reported causes of CTS, but it is not completely known how the process starts out or how it evolves for different people. Risk factors include age greater than 50, obesity, genetics (family history of CTS), gender (as it favors females over males), work type (highly-repetitive, hand-intensive work), pregnancy, birth control pill usage, thyroid disease, diabetes, rheumatoid arthritis, and more. In general, swelling is the culprit that results in pressure on the median nerve. This most commonly occurs from overuse of the hands and fingers. Playing musical instruments, sewing, crocheting, basket weaving, assembly/line work, meat processing work, typing/computer work, and waitressing are common over-use activities.

CLINICAL COURSE: Early into the disorder, CTS is usually easily managed and reversible. However, if the amount of pressure on the nerve is too much, the symptoms can become permanent. Think of a wire and how wearing away the plastic coating will "short" the wire. There are multiple layers to our nerves and the wearing away of the outer layers over time can become a problem resulting in permanent numbness and/or weakness.

BIGGEST MISTAKE: Don't wait until your symptoms are terrible! If you feel periodic numbness and tingling and you find yourself shaking your hand and "flicking" your fingers in attempt to "wake them up," NOW IS THE TIME TO COME VISIT YOUR CHIROPRACTOR before nerve damage occurs and the risk of permanency increases.

HOW CHIROPRACTIC HELPS: Treatment guidelines for CTS recommend a non-surgical approach, and this is where chiropractic comes in! A wrist night splint is typically recommended since sleep interruption due to numbness is

VERY common as we cannot control our wrist position when we sleep. Ice (not heat) is best as it reduces swelling (see #3 above). Rubbing an ice cube (or Dixie cup of ice) over the palm-side of the wrist works well. First, you will feel COLD followed by BURNING, then ACHING, and finally NUMBNESS ("C-BAN"). At this point STOP, as the next stage of cooling is frost bite! Do this three times a day or as directed. Your doctor of chiropractic will also talk to you about taking "mini-breaks" at home and/or at work and teach you exercises or stretches that can be performed during these breaks! A work station assessment is often very helpful as sometimes a simple change in work position or method can reduce wrist strain considerably. Your doctor of chiropractic may also perform manipulation to the small joints of the hand, wrist, elbow, shoulder, and neck as indicated in each specific case. He or she may also perform soft tissue release techniques to the muscles and soft tissues of the forearm, shoulder, and neck regions as needed. Surgery should be the LAST step in the treatment process, used only if all other non-surgical options have been tried without success.

The Challenges of Carpal Tunnel Syndrome

Carpal Tunnel Syndrome (CTS) is one of the most common "peripheral neuropathies" patients have when they visit a chiropractor for the first time. Peripheral neuropathy (PN) is defined as "…damage or disease affecting nerves, which may impair sensation, movement, gland or organ function, or other aspects of health, depending on the type of nerve affected." Let's take a closer look!

Common causes of PN include systemic conditions such as diabetes, vitamin deficiency, medication side effects (such as chemotherapy meds), traumatic injury, after radiation therapy, excessive alcohol intake, an autoimmune disease such as rheumatoid arthritis, and/or viral infection. PN can be linked to an individual's genetics that are present from birth. For others, it can be unknown which is then referred to as "idiopathic."

PN can affect one nerve (mononeuropathy) or multiple nerves (polyneuropathy) and can be acute (which means it comes on quickly) or chronic (which means it comes on gradually over time and progresses slowly). PN symptoms can include cramp/charley horse-like pain, muscle twitching, muscle atrophy or shrinkage, numbness, tingling, pins and needles, burning or cold feeling, and can also affect other tissues such as bone causing degeneration, skin changes, and hair and nail changes. PN can also affect a patient's balance and coordination which can increase an individual's chances of falling. If organs or glands are also impacted, PN can lead to poor bladder control, heart rate or blood pressure changes, and/or affect the sweat glands.

Getting back to CTS specifically, one of the challenges of this condition is determining the cause/s. Here's what we know about CTS: 1) it is more common in women than men; 2) it is more common in those who are overweight; 3) it is more common in those who work in highly repetitive environments; 4) it is more common over age 50; 5) it is often accompanied by other upper extremity "over-use" conditions like tendonitis in the hand, wrist, elbow, and/or shoulder and can also involve the neck (as CTS cases improve faster when treatment is also applied to the cervical spine); and 6) it commonly includes one or more of the conditions previously mentioned that can cause neuropathy such as diabetes and rheumatoid arthritis. Other conditions such as hypothyroid can also cause or worsen an existing case of CTS, in part due to "myxedema," a type of swelling that occurs with this condition. Here, the additional swelling can add to the compression or pressure pushing on the median nerve in the carpal tunnel and either cause CTS or worsen an existing case.

Because CTS can have more than one underlying cause, it's important that your doctor determine as many as possible in order to achieve the best treatment results. We've all heard of the cases that fail to respond to surgical intervention, which in many cases is because there were MULTIPLE CAUSES and only one was addressed with the surgical approach. Surgery has always been described as "the last resort" and indeed it's appropriate in some cases. However, MANY CTS patients respond well to chiropractic management, which often includes (but is not limited to): 1) joint manipulation and mobilization of the hand, wrist, forearm, elbow, shoulder, and neck; 2) use of a night-time splint; 3) home/work exercises; 4) physical therapy modalities; 5) nutritional considerations; and 6) ergonomic modifications (work station assessment). If these approaches fail to achieve satisfying results, your doctor will refer you to a hand surgeon to determine which procedure might be best for you.

Why Nighttime Pain with Carpal Tunnel Syndrome?

Chiropractors are often asked, "Why does Carpal Tunnel Syndrome (CTS) bother me so much during the night?" Let's take a look!

The carpal tunnel is made up of eight small carpal bones that bridge the forearm at the wrist would be very restricted and limited to bending a little bit up and a little bit down. Think of all the things you are able to do with a large range of motion at the wrist like tightening a small screw by hand, pulling on a wrench, using a hammer, working under the dash or inside the engine compartment of a car, threading a needle, sewing, knitting, crocheting, and even washing dishes. As you can see, we put our wrists in some pretty strange positions!

Look at the palm-side of your wrist and wiggle your fingers. Do you see all that activity going on? Now, move your eyes slowly towards the elbow as you keep moving your fingers. It is pretty amazing how much movement occurs near the elbow just by moving the fingers! There are actually nine tendons that travel through the carpal tunnel, and these tendons connect your forearm muscles to the fingers. That's why there is so much movement in the upper half of the forearm when moving your fingers, and in people with CTS, these muscles are usually overworked and super tight. This is why chiropractors work hard to loosen those muscles during treatment! These nine tendons are covered by a sheath, and friction between the tendon and the sheath is reduced by an oily substance called synovial fluid. When we repetitively and rapidly move our fingers, the friction that builds up produces heat, and if the oily synovial fluid can't keep up, swelling occurs.

Any situation where there is increased swelling in the body can also promote CTS. For example, during pregnancy, hormonal shifts can result in a generalized swelling similar to taking BCP's (birth control pills). Hypothyroid results in edema or swelling referred to as "myxedema" that can cause or make CTS worse. Some of the inflammatory arthritis conditions such as rheumatoid, lupus, scleroderma, and more can also predispose one to developing CTS. Obesity by itself is a risk factor for similar reasons.

So, why are we so susceptible to CTS symptoms at night? The main reason is that we RARELY sleep with our wrist in a straight or neutral position. We like to curl up in a fetal position and tuck our hands under our chin, bending the wrist to the full extent (90°). By doing so, the pressure inside the wrist "normally" doubles, but in the CTS patient, the pressure can increase by six times! This pinches the median nerve against the ligament that makes up the floor of the tunnel as it travels through the carpal tunnel, which then wakes us up and we find ourselves shaking and flicking our fingers to stop the numb, tingling, burning, pain that commonly occurs with CTS! This is why we prescribe a wrist brace for nighttime use and it REALLY helps! DON'T JUMP TO SURGERY FIRST – TRY CHIROPRACTIC FIRST!

The "Many Faces" of Carpal Tunnel Syndrome

Carpal Tunnel Syndrome (CTS) can present with a very mild, occasional numbness or tingling in the thumb, index, middle, and ring fingers and may never progress much beyond that point. But, for other patients, CTS is a painful, rapidly progressive problem that requires immediate attention. What makes it mild for some and bad for others? Let's take a look!

The common denominator of CTS is median nerve compression at the wrist resulting in the tingling, burning, itching in the palm, thumb, and fingers (except the little finger). Symptoms can also include weakness in grip strength, as the median nerve innervates muscles that help you grip things with your hands. The compression may occur from the nerve becoming swollen, inflammation of the surrounding tendons, a cyst forming in the tunnel (ganglion cyst is most common), and/or a bony spur from arthritis poking into the tunnel. There are other causes or "contributors" of CTS that may make it more intense for some than others. Fluid retention or edema can increase the pressure in the carpal tunnel. This can be caused by pregnancy, taking birth control pills, or by hormone replacement therapy (estrogen for osteoporosis and/or hot flashes). Another type of edema (called myxedema) is associated with low thyroid function, and CTS can be caused or worsened in those with hypothyroidism. Obesity is another risk factor for developing CTS. The shape of the wrist may also predispose some to CTS and when combined with other contributing causes, CTS symptoms may become quite severe. Trauma or injuries to the upper limb, especially fractures at the wrist, can cause CTS almost immediately, and an improperly treated wrist fracture (such as a colles fracture) can result in long-term CTS. Arthritis is often accelerated when wrist fractures occur and this can result in a long-term problem that includes stiffness in the joint with loss of movement and pain in addition to CTS signs and symptoms.

Another cause of CTS is diabetes. For diabetics, their blood can be thicker and have a more difficult time traveling through the small blood vessels (called capillaries) resulting in numbness and tingling of the distal extremities: the hands and feet. Over time, neuropathy creates a hypersensitivity of the nerve, and this can result in carpal tunnel syndrome and/or can make it more difficult to manage. It has also been reported that the use of insulin, metformin, as well as sulphonylureas, and thyroxine are associated with increased CTS management challenges. Over-activity of the pituitary gland (the "master gland") as it regulates the endocrine system is another contributor to CTS. Rheumatoid arthritis is a connective tissue disorder where antibodies inappropriately attack the lining of the joints creating swelling and pain. This can result in increased pressure on the median nerve in the carpal tunnel from both the inflamed joint as well as inflammation of the surrounding soft tissue. Combinations of these may also occur, which can make it challenging to determine which one(s) is the primary issue. Side effects to certain medications such as aromatase inhibitor drugs for breast cancer are also been well-published causes of CTS symptoms

The following activities have also been associated with an increased risk for CTS: vibrating hand tools, carrying heavy trays of food, working in a highly repetitive assembly-line type of job, milking cows, gardening, knitting, playing musical instruments, computer use, painting, meat and poultry processing, and carpentry.

Chiropractic offers a non-drug, non-surgical approach that is highly effective and therefore should be your FIRST STEP in the management of CTS!

Carpal Tunnel Syndrome: Onset and Symptoms

Carpal Tunnel Syndrome (CTS) is a painful, often debilitating, progressive condition that occurs when a nerve in the wrist becomes compressed. Let's take a closer look at what CTS is and what can be done for it!

ONSET: Often, CTS starts with an infrequent, vague sort of numbness or tingling that prompts us to periodically shake our hand and flick our fingers. Most of the time, we initially don't give this much thought, as it isn't too irritating. As time passes — and this can sometimes be days, weeks, or months — the intensity, frequency, and duration gradually worsen. Sooner or later, it can get to the point of prompting a visit to a Chiropractor. The rate that CTS progresses is more dependent on the amount of pressure on the median nerve more so than the length of time the pressure is applied. In other words, CTS can develop immediately if the nerve becomes acutely pinched from things like a wrist fracture or other obvious trauma. In these cases, it is VERY IMPORTANT that the nerve is decompressed promptly to avoid permanent nerve damage. However, a gradual worsening of symptoms over time is far more common, but it is still BEST to come in sooner rather than later since the greater the degree of inflammation or swelling, the longer the recovery time.

SYMPTOMS: The symptoms of CTS are quite unique and specific. It is not unusual for patients to say, "...I think I have carpal tunnel" when any complaint of the wrist or hand arises. CTS causes numbness, tingling, and/or pain specifically into the index, middle, and the thumb-side of the ring finger, as this is what the median nerve innervates, but not usually the thumb (unless the nerve is also compressed before the wrist). Numbness on the ring finger and pinky is usually the result of an ulnar nerve pinch, which frequently occurs at the inner elbow where the "funny bone" is located and/or at the shoulder ("thoracic outlet"), and/or the neck (from a pinched lower cervical nerve root). Combinations of these can result in a "double crush" or "multiple crush" injury and treatment must then focus on ALL the places where the nerve compression occurs. This is why you should consider obtaining CTS treatment sooner rather than later, because when you wait and let it go, the tendency is to start making changes in the way you use your arms and hands. This is an unconscious compensatory response that often leads to further problems higher up in the arm and/or neck.

According to the National Institute of Neurological Disorders and Stroke, CTS is the MOST COMMON of the "entrapment neuropathies" where the body's peripheral nerves become compressed or pinched. It is estimated that 5% of women and

3% of men have CTS, and studies estimate 3-6% of adults (most commonly between ages 45-64 years) in the general population suffer from CTS. Chiropractic offers a non-drug, non-surgical approach that is highly effective. This should be your FIRST STEP in treatment as surgery can often be avoided!

7 Possible Causes of Carpal Tunnel Syndrome

Carpal Tunnel Syndrome (CTS) is a condition caused by compression of the median nerve as it travels through the carpal tunnel at the wrist, possibly resulting in numbness, tingling, and eventually weakness in the thumb and the index, middle, and ring fingers. "True" CTS occurs when the median nerve is pinched while it travels through the carpal tunnel; however, other conditions can mimic and/or contribute to CTS. Let's take a look at seven possible causes of CTS...

1. Swelling of the flexor tendons: This is probably the most common cause of carpal tunnel symptoms and is usually due to overuse of the hands associated with highly repetitive tasks like line work, computer typing, sewing, knitting, or playing a musical instrument. When fast repetitive gripping is required, especially if firm gripping is needed and/or the environment is cold, symptoms can occur more quickly. There is a sheath that wraps around the tendons traveling through the tunnel that is lubricated by synovial fluid. This normally keeps the tendon sliding freely inside the sheath. In the CTS patient, the tendon and/or the sheath tightens and creates swelling as extra synovial fluid is produced in an attempt to remedy the excess friction. This increases the pressure inside the sheath and causes more swelling and pain, and eventually conditions such as tendonitis and/or tenosynovitis. If left untreated, this can result in "trigger finger" (stenosing tenosynovitis) that can be more resistant to treatment. This enlarged, swollen tendon-sheath complex places pressure upon the median nerve and results in the classic symptoms of CTS.

94

2. Misalignment of carpal bones: If one or more of the eight carpal bones become misaligned, it can cause the transverse carpal ligament (the floor of the tunnel) to tighten, narrowing the carpal tunnel and compressing it contents — including the median nerve!
3. Direct compression of the tunnel: ANY occupation that requires the use of hand tools or any other objects that apply pressure directly to the carpal tunnel can cause CTS. Examples include hammers, screwdrivers, drills, pliers, jackhammers, a computer mouse, and more.
4. Vibration: Any job or tool that requires firm gripping and vibration such as jackhammers, chain saws, hand buffers, or grinders can irritate the contents inside the carpal tunnel.
5. Cold Temperatures: Cold vasoconstricts blood vessels and decreases blood flow to the area. When the cold exposure is prolonged, the lack of blood flow can keep needed oxygen from reaching the tissues that need it, possibly causing injury or contributing to an existing injury. Meatpacking or poultry plants are good examples of jobs requiring highly repetitive work in a cold environment.
6. Arthritis: Old injuries (such as wrist fractures) or jobs that wear down the hyaline cartilage (smooth covering on joints) over time can result in spurs that can compress the nerve. Inflammatory arthritis, like rheumatoid, can also add pressure to the tunnel resulting in CTS.
7. Multiple crush: More than one compression location on the median nerve can worsen CTS. This added compression can occur at the forearm, elbow, shoulder, and / or neck.

Carpal Tunnel Syndrome "Home Remedies"

Carpal Tunnel Syndrome (CTS) results in pain, numbness, tingling, grip strength weakness, interrupted sleep, and can interfere with work, social family, and recreational activities. Symptoms can radiate up the forearm and into the fingers making tasks that require intricate finger movements very difficult. Many of us know someone who has had carpal tunnel surgery, but what can be done in order to avoid surgery? Let's find out!

Exercise : The follow five exercises should be performed MANY times a day! The goals are to keep the tendons traveling through the carpal tunnel freely, promote better circulation, remove the pinch on the median nerve, and strengthen muscles. As a general warning, modify or STOP ANY exercise if you feel sharp pain or worsening of symptoms!

1. WRIST CIRCLES: Palms down, elbows bent 90 degrees, draw a circle with your third/long finger. Repeat five times, clockwise and counterclockwise. Increase the size of the circle with each repetition.
2. THUMB STRETCH: Place the palm of your hand on a wall (elbow straight) fingers pointing downward. Reach across and pull your thumb back and hold for five seconds and repeat three to five times.
3. 5-FINGER STRETCH/"BEAR CLAW"/FIST: a) Spread your fingers out of both hands as far as possible; b) Bend ONLY the fingers tips (not your big knuckle joints); c) Make a tight fist. HOLD each position for five seconds repeat three to five times.
4. WRIST CURLS (4 positions: Palm up, Thumb up, Palm down, Pinky up): Using either Thera-Band / Tubing or light hand weights, sit and rest your forearm on your thigh; position your hand palm up and lift the weight/stretch the tubing towards the ceiling. SLOWLY release the resistance on the tubing / lower the weight towards the floor. Repeat this three to five times in each of the four hand positions listed above. For the "pinky up" exercise, raise your arm from your side so you can position your hand so the pinky faces the ceiling. Feel free to support your wrist with your other hand. You can gradually increase the weight (max. 5 lbs./2.27 kg) / band resistance.
5. NECK STRETCHES: Bend your head sideways to the right and reach over with the right hand and pull gently while reaching down towards the ground with the left. Move your head and neck into various positions feeling

for a good stretch in different tight neck muscles. Repeat this on the other side.

Diet and Nutrition : This is very important, as you can reduce the inflammatory markers in your body quite well by doing some very simple things! First, stop eating grains, as they can cause inflammation! Supplement your diet with 4000 IU of fish oil / day and 5000IU of vitamin D3 per day (of course, talk with your Doctor first). Avoid sugar as much as possible. This will not only help reduce your swelling, but usually boosts your energy and helps with weigh loss – as obesity is a risk factor for CTS!
Sleep : Since we cannot control the position of our wrist when sleeping, wearing a splint that holds your wrist straight at night is extremely helpful. We will help you with this!

Driving : It's common for CTS symptoms to worsen while you hold the steering wheel. Position your hands at an 8 and 4 o'clock position on the wheel to keep the wrist straight. Wearing the splints when driving can help as well.

Chiropractic Care : There are often multiple sites between the neck (where the median nerve starts) and wrist that needs to be kept loose to minimize nerve compression. These treatments are very effective for many people!

Carpal Tunnel Syndrome During Pregnancy

While Carpal Tunnel Syndrome (CTS) is usually characterized as a repetitive stress injury, it can also be caused by pregnancy. In fact, CTS is a common complaint among pregnant women due to the increase in fluid build-up in the tissues, including the forearms and wrist. Edema is the technical term for fluid build-up, and it is hard to avoid during pregnancy. This swelling results in increased pressure on the median nerve that originates in the neck, travels through the shoulder, into the arm, through the wrist and innervates the thumb, index, third and half of the fourth finger. The "usual" initial symptoms include a "half-asleep" sensation in the fingertips prompting the sufferer to shake and "flick" the fingers in attempt to "…wake them up." These symptoms (with or without pregnancy) commonly occur at night, as many tend to sleep with wrists in bent positions. When we bend our wrist in any direction, the pressure inside the carpal tunnel will double.

This can happen even more if there is edema or swelling present from the hormonal shift that occurs during pregnancy. This is why chiropractors will frequently fit CTS patients with a "cock up splint," which is to be used primarily at night, as it often gets in the way during routine daytime activities. However, there may be times when the cock-up splint can be quite beneficial, such as when driving and holding onto the steering wheel. Grip strength may also be affected, making buttoning shirts and opening jars difficult. CTS may only affect your dominant hand, but it can affect both. It is less common that CTS only impacts the non-dominant hand. There is an increased likelihood of developing CTS if you had it previously and/or if other family members have had CTS. Also, if you've had problems with your neck, back, or shoulder, such as an old whiplash injury, slipped disk in the neck, or broken collar bone, you are also at greater risk of developing CTS. If you were obese before the pregnancy and/or put on too much weight during the pregnancy, this too will increase the risk.

Besides the splint, other forms of care during pregnancy include: 1) EAT A BALANCED DIET. Include small amounts of lean protein (meat, poultry, eggs, beans) with each meal. Reduce the amount of salt, sugar, and fat you eat and drink PLENTY OF WATER! Eat at least five portions of fruit and veggies EVERY DAY! 2) VITAMIN B6. Pyridoxine or B6 has been reported to help CTS sufferers, and it is good for the nervous system. Foods rich in B6 include sunflower and sesame seeds, dark green vegetables (like broccoli), garlic, hazelnuts, lean meat, avocados, and fish (salmon and cod especially). Consider a B6 supplement, but DON'T exceed 150mg/day. 3) MATERNITY BRA. Be sure to wear a good fitting maternity bra with straps that don't dig into your shoulders and neck. Wear it early on, as this can reduce the weight off your neck, ribcage, and shoulders and can help avoid compression of the median nerve. 4) Herbs such as chamomile tea, ginger, turmeric, and others that fight inflammation can be effective – we will guide you on the dose! 5) Wrist exercises, wrist manipulation/mobilization, traction, and muscle release work can ALL be VERY effective which we can provide for you .

Repeat these two exercises on BOTH sides so you can feel the difference between the two, regardless if you have problems on both sides. Since the neck and shoulder can be involved, we will also show you how to stretch these areas, as keeping the whole "kinetic chain" stretched is very important for long-term benefits.

Carpal Tunnel Syndrome – What Can I Do to Help? (Part 1)

Carpal Tunnel Syndrome (CTS) can arise as a result of a number of different causes and as such, treatment is guided by the specific needs of the individual and tailored to each individual case. With that said, there are specific treatment strategies that chiropractors provide that address three primary goals: 1) Physical management strategies; 2) Chemical management strategies; and 3) Self-management strategies. All three goals include a component that we, the doctor, control AND a component that you, the patient, can control or manage. This combined effort or "team approach" ALWAYS works best, especially over the long-term. So, let's break these three management strategies down along with the two components: my job (as your chiropractor) and your job (as my patient)!

1) Physical management strategies : This category addresses the mechanical nature of CTS. That is, compression of the median nerve at ALL of the possible sites, not JUST the wrist/carpal tunnel area. Since the median nerve arises initially from the neck or cervical spine, nerve root compression of C6-T1 (and a little of C5) can give rise to CTS signs and symptoms. As

discussed last month, this area can be one of the "great imposters" of CTS and/or it may contribute as a co-conspirator and combine with CTS, which magnifies or increases the CTS signs and symptoms, the so-called "double-crush syndrome." Other "mechanical" sites of compression can be reviewed in last month's Health Update, but in brief, these may include the thoracic outlet (shoulder area), Struther's ligament (just above the elbow), the pronator tunnel (just below the elbow), the anterior interosseous membrane (forearm), as well as at the carpal tunnel itself.

MY JOB (as your chiropractor) is to reduce the pressure on the nerve at any and/or ALL these locations (remember, each case is unique). This can be done by using manual therapies including (but not limited to) manipulation of joints in the neck, shoulder, arm, elbow, forearm, wrist, hand, and fingers. Mobilization of muscles and other soft tissues may include active release techniques, friction massage, trigger point therapy, stretching with and without resistance, traction, and more. Various modalities might be used to reduce muscle tightness, swelling, or inflammation.

A nighttime wrist splint keeps the wrist in a neutral position, as the carpal tunnel's pressure goes up A LOT when the wrist is bent. Since you cannot control the position of your wrist while you sleep, the brace can REALLY HELP! A BIG part of my job includes teaching YOU about CTS so that you understand the underlying causes, thus allowing you to identify jobs, hobbies, or situations where you may be inadvertently harming yourself. If you can, PROMPTLY identify offending wrist positions and STOP the repetitive injurious movement and then MODIFY your approach to the task, whether it means taking "mini-breaks," changing the work station set up, or some other approach. Along with this "teaching concept" is exercise training. It is also VERY IMPORTANT for you to properly perform the carpal tunnel stretches and other exercises (see Part 2 next month) on a regimented/regular basis.

YOUR JOB includes wearing the brace (don't forget or procrastinate), most importantly at night. You can wear it during the day while driving or doing something where you are not "fighting" the brace. In some cases, the brace can bruise you if you are moving your wrist against it repetitively or too hard, and it can actually do more harm than good in those situations. Your job is also to identify ways to do your job and/or hobbies with less torque or twisting of your wrist.

Next month's discussion will start chemical strategies (#2 on the list above), which includes several very effective and safe approaches in the CTS management process. We will then address #3, "Self-management strategies," which will include various CTS-specific exercises.

Carpal Tunnel Syndrome – What Can I Do to Help? (Part 2)

Carpal Tunnel Syndrome (CTS) management strategies were introduced last month, which we will conclude this month with Part 2. In part one, we cited three primary goals of CTS management that include the following: 1) Physical management strategies; 2) Chemical management strategies; and 3) Self-management strategies. All three goals include a component that we as doctors of chiropractic control AND (most important), a component that you the patient controls. We will continue this discussion this month with chemical management strategies.

2. Chemical management strategies : Here, MY JOB includes guiding you in methods to reduce swelling or inflammation. The first method involves the use of ice. Different cooling approaches include the use of ice cup/massage (applied directly on the skin until numb, which takes about five minutes) and/or ice packs (takes about 10-15 minutes). We can also offer assistance in choosing various anti-inflammatory herbs (such as ginger, tumeric, boswellia) and vitamins (such as vitamin B6 or

pyridoxine; magnesium, fish oil / omega 3 fatty acids, vitamin D) with anti-inflammatory properties. Recently, probiotics have also been demonstrated to reduce inflammation! YOUR JOB is to follow these recommendations that you and I agree upon to help reduce the inflammatory effects of CTS. Other "chemical strategies" may include adding the primary care physician to "the team," as prescriptions for various conditions such as diabetes, hypothyroidism, rheumatoid arthritis, and others may be appropriate in certain CTS cases.

3) Self-management strategies : Though we have already looked at "MY JOB" and "YOUR JOB" as it pertains to 1) Physical management and 2) Chemical management strategies, overlap exists between all three CTS management goals. In other words, as the name implies, "self-management strategies" includes the need for you to comply with the recommendations. For example, wearing the cock-up wrist splint primarily at night (when sleeping and less commonly at times during the day), following instructions regarding job modifications, nutritional strategies and, when applicable, pharmaceutical intervention are things you can do to alleviate symptoms. One of the MOST IMPORTANT self-help strategies is the training of carpal tunnel specific exercises, as well as exercise in general. Maintaining a proper weight (a BMI between 20-25) is also a goal that will help CTS, as obesity is a risk factor for this condition and a host of other conditions, including diabetes!

EXERCISE #1 : Stand near a wall. Place your palm on the wall at shoulder height pointing the fingers down towards the floor, keeping the elbow straight. Reach across with the opposite hand and pull your thumb back as you stretch the palm-side forearm muscles. Hold 5-10 seconds until you feel the muscle "melt." Repeat three times per side, five times a day. You can use the edge of a counter top rather than a wall, if you like.

EXERCISE #2 : Bend the elbow 90 degrees. "Dig" your thumb DEEP into the palm-side forearm muscles close to the elbow. Slowly straighten the elbow and maintain the deep pressure into the muscle until the elbow is completely straight. REPEAT this multiple times moving your thumb one inch closer to your wrist from the last pressure point until you are one to two inches from the wrist (or, until you don't feel much tenderness). You can vary the speed at which you straighten the elbow but generally, slower is better than fast movement, and the deeper the pressure, the better.

Repeat these two exercises on BOTH sides so you can feel the difference between the two, regardless if you have problems on both sides. Since the neck and shoulder can be involved, we will also show you how to stretch these areas, as keeping the whole "kinetic chain" stretched is very important for long-term benefits.

Great Imposters of Carpal Tunnel Syndrome

Carpal Tunnel Syndrome (CTS) is caused by compression and subsequent irritation of the median nerve as it travels through the carpal tunnel and into the hand where it innervates the palm side of the second to fourth digits. As stated last month, the median nerve is sometimes referred to as, "...the eye of the hand" since we rely so heavily on activities of daily living (ADLs) that require its health and function. Some of these ADLs include buttoning a shirt, picking up small objects, tying a shoe or neck tie, writing, holding a book or coffee cup, gripping items such as a phone or steering wheel, opening jars, household chores, and carrying objects, especially with the finger tips.

When patients present with CTS signs and symptoms, one would think that the examination and treatment would be fairly straightforward and "routine." The problem is, no two cases of CTS are identical because of all the possible mitigating factors, or the presence of OTHER issues that may be contributing or may be the REAL cause for CTS in that particular person. This may explain the reason surgical release of the transverse carpal ligament doesn't always work!

The "Great Imposters" of CTS include both physical and chemical factors. Physical factors include (but are not limited to): 1) Cervical nerve root compression: Since the median nerve originates from the C6-T1 (and a little from C5) nerve roots exiting the spine, it only makes sense that a pinched nerve in the neck can mimic a pinched nerve at the wrist. The difference here is "usually" that the whole arm is involved, which is less likely in CTS only. Moving down from the neck, the next most common location for a mechanical pinch is at the 2) Thoracic outlet: Here, the nerve roots coming from C5 to T2, like merging lanes of a highway, come together to make the three main nerves that enter the arm and along with the blood vessels, this "neurovascular bundle" leaves the upper chest region and travels through the thoracic outlet to enter into the arm. The thoracic outlet can become narrowed if there is an extra rib, a shift in the collar bone or shoulder blade, from muscles that are too tight (especially the anterior scalene and/or pectoralis minor), or from anything that occupies space within the thoracic outlet. 3) Struther's ligament: In a few of us (only about 2%), there is a ligament just above the elbow that can entrap the median (as well as the ulnar) nerve, creating a pinch and subsequent numbness below that point, mimicking CTS. 4) Pronator tunnel: The median nerve is more commonly entrapped by the pronator teres muscle just below the elbow, and treating this location can be highly rewarding when managing stubborn CTS cases. Less common is entrapment in the mid-forearm, though it's possible by either the interosseous membrane that connects the ulna and radius or from fracture of the ulna and/or radius. The most distal point of median nerve compression is at the carpal tunnel. Entrapments can be singular or multiple and when more than one "tunnel" compresses the median nerve, the term double or multiple crush is utilized. Management MUST address ALL points of compression to obtain long-term satisfying results. Other "imposters" of CTS include a host of conditions including (but not limited to) thyroid disease, diabetes, arthritis, pregnancy, birth control pill use, obesity, and MANY others! Chiropractic makes the most sense when it comes to managing CTS from mechanical causes. If response is slow or not satisfying, we will

104

order tests and/or consults to get to the bottom of what "imposters" may be contributing to your CTS symptoms!

Carpal Tunnel Syndrome – What Is It?

Carpal Tunnel Syndrome (CTS) basically occurs when pressure is applied to the median nerve as it travels through the wrist on the palm side resulting in numbness, tingling, pain, and later, weakness of the grip and pinch functions. But, the median nerve can be pinched at many other locations as it courses down from the neck to the hand, which is why we examine and treat the CTS patient from the neck down! The median nerve has been described as the "eye of the hand," as it is one of the three major nerves formed from the brachial plexus—that "highway" of nerves made up of the C5-T2 roots leaving the neck, merging together to eventually form the three main nerves of the arm. Because the median nerve function regulates pinch and grip strength, buttoning a shirt, writing a note, driving a car, and even sleeping are ALL affected by a median nerve pinch. But WHAT is CTS? Let's take an "inside" look!

We know that fast, repetitive motion-related jobs like meat or fish packing plants, assembly line work, sewing occupations, and the like can cause CTS over time. Look at the palm side of your wrist and wiggle your fingers. Do you see ALL THE MOVEMENT that is occurring just before the wrist in the forearm? That motion is coming from the tendons, which like shoe strings, attach the forearm muscles to the fingers. Notice ALL the movement in your forearm muscles closer to the elbow – that's a lot of motion! There are nine tendons that are covered by a lubricating sheath that help the fast moving tendons reduce friction, thus decreasing the chances for heat build up, swelling (inflammation), and subsequent pain and loss of function. But, there is a limit or threshold that the tendons and sheaths can withstand before they just can't keep up. These nine tendons and sheaths are quite tightly packed together as they leave the forearm and enter the carpal tunnel.

The carpal tunnel is made up of eight small wrist bones called the "carpal bones," and ANYTHING that makes that tunnel more narrow can effectively cause CTS. If we look at what happens INSIDE the tunnel in the CTS patient, the venous blood flow and nerve flow (called "axonal transport") is blocked when the PRESSURE inside the tunnel occurs. We all know what it feels like when a blood pressure cuff is inflated on our arm – if it's pumped up too high or left on too long, the arm REALLY HURTS! That's because the blood can't get past the inflated cuff and oxygen can't get to our muscles and tissues past the cuff and IT CAUSES PAIN!

To give you an appreciation of the pressure difference between the normal vs. CTS wrist, normally, the pressure ranges between 2 and 10 mmHg. We pump up a blood pressure cuff to about 150-200 mmHg when we take blood pressure, so this is NOT MUCH! This 2-10 mmHg pressure increases when we change the position of our fingers, wrist and forearm with wrist extension (bending the hand backwards), causing the greatest pressure increase. This is why we fit the CTS patient with a wrist "cock-up" splint to be worn at night since you can't control your wrist position when you sleep and any bent position increases the pressure and can wake you up due to numbness, tingling, pain prompting you to shake and flick your hands and fingers until they, "...wake up." When CTS is present, the pressure inside the tunnel goes up exponentially, meaning NOT 2 or 3 times, but 6, 12, 24 times what is normal and even higher! Now, if you add wrist bending (extension > flexion), the pressure REALLY gets high and it doesn't take long for the nerve pinch and blood loss to wake us up. We've previously talked about other conditions that can make developing CTS more common or make it worse like hypothyroid, diabetes, arthritis, kidney disease, and more. AGAIN, this is because an increase is pressure results from these conditions (increased swelling = increased pressure = increased symptoms). As chiropractors, we will guide and manage your care through the healing process of CTS using a conservative, NON-SURGICAL treatment approach – TRY THIS FIRST!

Carpal Tunnel Syndrome and the Neck?

Carpal Tunnel Syndrome (CTS) is a problem that occurs when the median nerve gets pinched as it passes through the tunnel at the wrist, resulting in numbness that includes the palm side of the hand, the thumb through digit three and the thumb-side half of the ring or fourth finger. So, how does the neck fit into the cause and/or the treatment of CTS? Let's take a look!

The neck is comprised of seven vertebrae and eight pairs of nerves that travel down the arms allowing us to feel sensations such as hot/cold, vibration, and sharp/dull. These nerves allow us to move our muscles and joints including the fingers, wrist, elbow and shoulder. These eight pairs of nerve roots, like a super highway of eight lanes of traffic, eventually merge into the ulnar, median, and radial nerves that extend down our arms. The median nerve is the primary nerve involved in carpal tunnel syndrome, so let's take a look at the route that it takes as it leaves the cervical spine, or neck.

Initially, when the eight nerve roots first exit the spine they interconnect forming the brachial plexus, and by the time the nerves reach the arm pit, they've "merged" into the three main nerves that extend the rest of the way down the arm. The median nerve can become trapped or pinched at a number of different places, most commonly at the wrist's carpal tunnel followed by the pronator tunnel which is located at the elbow just past the crease on the palm side. It can also be pinched before the elbow by a ligament that exists in about 1% of us (Struther's Ligament), but this is rare.

If a fracture should occur anywhere along the route of the nerve, that too can cause a compression. The neck is a common location where the cause of the numbness can arise. The median nerve arises from three nerve roots that exit the neck (C5, C6, and C7); therefore, ANYTHING that places pressure at this location in the neck can result in similar symptoms as CTS.

The term, "double crush" syndrome applies to the situation where compression (pinching) of a nerve occurs in more than one place. This was first discussed in 1973 and has since been a debated topic. When a nerve is compressed in more than one location, there is a physiological change in the way the nerve transmits a signal and a minor (sub-clinical) compression that would by itself not be symptom-producing becomes symptomatic if a second compression occurs elsewhere along the course of the nerve. Similarly, metabolic changes, such as diabetes, can also make minor CTS symptomatic. This is why it is ESSENTIAL that the entire course of the nerve be tested, not just at the wrist but also at the neck, shoulder, and arm. I'm sure you can see the importance of this, as surgical decompression at the wrist may NOT help in a case where a more significant pinch is present elsewhere. This has been estimated to occur between 30-75% of the time! A common site for double crush with CTS is at the cervical nerve root, and treatment of the compression site in the neck by a chiropractic adjustment can MAKE OR BREAK a successful outcome when treating CTS. The bottom line? Try chiropractic FIRST as you can't reverse an unnecessary surgery!

Carpal Tunnel Treatment Options

The goal of any treatment approach for Carpal Tunnel Syndrome (CTS) is to return the patient to normal. That means addressing all OTHER health related conditions that can cause CTS such as diabetes, hypothyroidism, birth control pill use, pregnancy, rheumatoid arthritis (and many of the other related arthritic-like disorders), as well as double or multiple crush (pinched nerve) syndromes. That's right! CTS can be caused by MANY other conditions besides simply overusing the arms and hands. When overuse PLUS any of the above mentioned conditions "gang-up" on you, managing BOTH is necessary.

One "universal" goal in CTS treatment is to reduce inflammation. This can be accomplished by several approaches: 1) STOP, reduce, and/or modify the causing activity. Examples include repetitive use of a hammer, screw driver, stapler, assembly line work, typing/computer work, driving with a firm grip on the steering wheel, bicycle riding, and MANY more! The key to successful management of CTS is to slow down, stop/rest, and for long-term success, change how the task is performed (modify the work station). 2) Wearing a cock-up wrist splint. This is usually restricted to night time use since we cannot control our wrist position while sleeping and the pressure inside the carpal tunnel "normally" doubles at the extremes of the wrist forwards or backwards. Thus, keeping the wrist straight at night significantly reduces or eliminates the numbness/tingling that can cause multiple sleep interruptions. It can also be worn during the day IF it doesn't interfere with the person's activity. If the activity requires frequent bending of the wrist, you'll end up fighting against the wrist splint and that can actually worsen your CTS! 3) Ice cupping or massage. Freeze water in a Styrofoam or paper Dixie cup (like home-made popsicles) and peel away the top third to expose the ice. Rub it over the palm side of the wrist until you feel numbness. At first, it will feel C old, followed by B urning, A ching, and finally N umbness (hence the acronym, "C-BAN"). The length of time to achieve numbness is usually three to five minutes, but make sure you quit at the point of numbness as the next stage is frostbite! 4) Anti-inflammatory nutrients. An anti-inflammatory diet is one that is rich in fruits, vegetables, lean meats, omega-3 fatty acids, and avoids glutens, omega-6 fatty acids (fast foods, etc.), and refined carbohydrates (sweets, sodas, etc.). Also, there are many REALLY GOOD nutritional supplements that can effectively reduce inflammation without the typical side-effects that affect the stomach, liver, or kidneys which are common to NSAID drugs like aspirin, ibuprofen, or Aleve. Also, NSAIDs can inhibit an important chemical (a prostaglandin) that is needed for healing, and therefore, it can actually slow down the healing process (so try the nutritional approaches first)! Nutritional options include proteolytic enzymes, Bromelain, papain, bioflavonoid, Vitamin C, Vitamin D, Vitamin E, Coenzyme Q10, and many more.

Treatment options beyond those mentioned above are typically surgical, IF you decide to go to a surgeon. However, chiropractic care includes identifying and treating the source(s) of nerve irritation, as it is often more than just nerve pinching at the carpal tunnel. Other common locations of median nerve entrapment includes the pronator teres muscle in the forearm just past the elbow on the palm side, less often at the shoulder, and again quite frequently in the neck where the nerve exits the spine. If these areas of nerve pinching are not released, recovery is less likely (with or without surgery)! Bottom line, you can always have surgery but you can't "un-do it." Try chiropractic first as it's the least invasive, least costly, and often the quickest way to find relief from CTS!

CTS Self-Diagnosis – Is That Possible?

Carpal Tunnel Syndrome (CTS) is technically a "pinched nerve" in the wrist (carpal tunnel) that results in numbness, tingling and later, weakness in the distribution of the median nerve (thumb, index, 3rd, and half of the 4th finger). There is a limited amount of space within the carpal tunnel. In addition to the median nerve, there are 9 tendons and their sheaths, a network of blood vessels, the joint capsules, the bony "roof" and ligamentous "floor." Any condition that distorts the shape of the tunnel (inflammatory conditions like rheumatoid arthritis, ganglion cysts, bony spurs, or conditions that result in swelling like overuse, pregnancy, taking birth control pills, hypothyroid, obesity, and/or conditions that create neuropathy like a pinched nerve in the neck, shoulder or elbow, diabetes and post-chemotherapy) can result in median nerve irritation. The carpal tunnel naturally changes its shape when we flex and extend the wrist, so occupations that require wrist bending (especially if it's prolonged and a fast pace is required) such as carpentry (especially the use of vibrating tools), waitressing, assembly line work, typists, and even sleeping at night with the wrist bent can result in CTS.

110

The diagnosis can be tricky because of all the possible causes (of which, some are described above) and to make matters even more challenging, there can be two, three, or more of the causes all contributing to the problem at the same time! In the clinic, there are certain positions to test how long (in seconds) it takes for the numbness, tingling and/or pain to occur when we place the wrist in extreme flexion or extension. We'll compress the carpal tunnel (and nerve pathways at the elbow, shoulder, and neck), as well as tap over the carpal tunnel with a reflex hammer creating a "funny bone" sensation usually into the 2nd or 3rd finger. Blood tests for rheumatoid (and other inflammatory) arthritis, diabetes and thyroid dysfunction are very helpful when trying to differentiate between several possible causes. An electrical conduction test called electromyogram (EMG) and nerve conduction velocity (NCV) can also be very helpful in determining the severity of CTS.

So the question is, can you "self-diagnose" CTS? The answer is: sometimes. However, with that said, if the symptoms are "classic" (numbness/tingling in the thumb, fingers 2-4, which shaking and flicking your fingers relieves at least partially; it's waking you up at night especially, if a night splint helps reduce the frequency of waking and intensity of numbness), then you "probably" have CTS. Here are some common questions included in a CTS questionnaire that we often use in the clinic to assist with the diagnosis: SYMPTOM SEVERITY (score each on a 0-4 scale): 1) Pain severity at night? 2) Nighttime frequency of waking with pain? 3) Amount of daytime hand/wrist pain? 4) Frequency of daytime hand/wrist pain? 5) Duration (in minutes) of daytime pain/numbness? 6) Severity of numbness? 7) Severity of weakness? 8) Tingling intensity? 9) Nighttime severity of numbness or tingling? 10) Nighttime frequency of numbness or tingling? 11) Difficulty grasping / using small objects like keys or pens? FUNCTION SEVERITY (0-4 scale): 1) Writing. 2) Buttoning clothes. 3) Holding a book while reading. 4. Gripping of a telephone handle. 5) Opening jars. 6. Household chores. 7. Carrying grocery bags. 8. Bathing and dressing. The maximum score for SYMPTOM SEVERITY is 11x4 = 44 and for

FUNCTION 8x4 = 32. To determine the percentage, divide your score by 76 (the maximum possible) and multiply it by 100. In general, scores >50% may be indicative of CTS. However, as previously stated, a definitive diagnosis must include a detailed history, examination, sometimes special tests. Therefore, it is important to see us! If you have CTS, we will outline the type and length of care with you and MOST IMPORTANT, we can usually manage CTS without the need for surgery!

Carpal Tunnel Syndrome – Nutritional Considerations

Carpal Tunnel Syndrome (CTS) is a condition where the median nerve that arises in the neck and travels through the shoulder, arm, and into the hand becomes compressed. Compression of the median nerve results in tingling, numbness, pain and/or weakness that affects the 2nd, 3rd, and thumb-side half of the 4th fingers. It can wake sufferers up in the middle of the night, forcing them to have to shake the hand and flick the fingers to "wake it up." This can occur multiples times a night, making for a long next day! We've discussed chiropractic management strategies such as manipulation/mobilization of the neck, shoulder, elbow, wrist and hand, the use of a cock-up splint (especially at night and at times when driving), but more information regarding the use of nutritional supplementation is lacking; hence the purpose of this Health Update!

Let's look at what we are trying to accomplish by

1. Anti-inflammation : Because of stomach, liver, and kidney side effects, NSAIDs such as ibuprofen, aspirin, and others may not be your best choice. Rather, consider Turmeric (300 mcg), Ginger (100 mg), Boswellia (100 mg), Rosemary (100 mg), Bioflavonoid (100 mg), Bromelain (50 mg), Vitamin C (1-3 grams/day), Vitamin E (400 IU/day), Vitamin D3 (2000-5000 IU/day), Vitamin B-complex (especially B6, 9, and 12).

2. Muscle relaxation : Calcium (1500mg/day), Magnesium (400 mg/day), Potassium, valerian root (vervain), B-Complex, L-Arginine, Rosemary, Catnip, Kava root, Chamomile, Cayenne Pepper, Horseradish, Lavender, Licorice, Devil's Claw.

3. Nerve repair : Folate (B9), B12 (cobalamin), Vitamin D3, B1 (Thiamin; minimum: 1.2mg/day), B5 (Pantothenic acid), B3 (niacin; minimum 16 mg/day), B12.

4. Managing systemic conditions :

Diabetes (dysinsulinism) : Chromium (picolinate or choloride), Alpha-Lipoic Acid, Omega-3 Fatty Acids (1000 mg of EPA & DHA), Coenzyme Q10, Polyphenols (dark chocolate, green tea), Botanicals (plant extracts such as garlic, prickly pear, aloe vera, fenugreek, bitter melon and ginseng).

- Thyroid dysfunction (hypothyroid) : B-Complex (100 mg of B1, 3, 5, & 6 3x/day; B2, 50 mg 2x/day; B12 1000-2000 mcg/day; Selenium and iodine, Anti-oxidants (Selenium, Vit. C, Vit. E) Copper, thyroid extract, organic iodine.
- Obesity (BMI>30) : Childhood obesity: Vit. D (ages 1-13, 5 mcg/day), B12, Vit. C, Fiber, Calcium (an extra 300mg of Calcium= >2 lb. weight drop); other fat soluble vitamins (Vit. A, E, and K), iron (iron is more commonly deficient in obese children and adults and can lead to fatigue and poor mental health and memory function).

5. Other considerations : General health: paleo diet, sleep quality, and exercise (see below).

You may notice that there is a lot of overlap in many of these vitamin recommendations. If one were to give nutritional recommendations for general health purposes, the anti-inflammatory "big 5" might include 1. A good quality multi-vitamin mineral, 2. Magnesium (often with calcium as a combined supplement), 3. Omega-3 fatty acids; 4. Vitamin D; and 5. Coenzyme Q10. For CTS specifically, the addition of a B complex seems consistently recommended above. Controlling weight will reduce CTS risk and decrease the risk of acquiring type II diabetes which increases CTS risk by itself. Perhaps an "ideal diet" for everyone might include eating plenty of fruits, vegetables, lean meats, and the elimination of gluten (grains) – referred to by some as the "anti-inflammatory diet," paleo diet, caveman diet, and Mediterranean diet. Fortifying a great diet with vitamins is the "take-home" concept!

Carpal Tunnel Syndrome vs. A Pinched Nerve Elsewhere

Carpal Tunnel Syndrome (CTS) is a common complaint presented to chiropractic offices. Usually, patients wait for weeks, months, or even years before seeking care, thus making management more challenging. The history of the "classic" CTS patient includes a mild, sporadic onset that gradually becomes more frequent and intense. This usually leads to continued problems that start to affect other areas proximal to the hand, such as the elbow, shoulder and/or neck. We usually find that people will compensate during their activities, and instead of moving the wrist and hand to perform a task, they will start to move their elbow and shoulder more to avoid irritating movements of the hand/wrist. Over time, overloading the muscles in these areas can lead to one or more conditions commonly referred to as "cumulative trauma disorder" (CTD), which includes many diagnoses including (but not limited to) tendonitis of the thumb (de Quervain's Disease), ganglion cysts, tennis elbow (lateral epicondylitis), golfer's or bowler's elbow (medial epicondylitis), cubital tunnel syndrome (ulnar nerve pinch at the medial elbow), tunnel of Guyon syndrome (ulnar nerve pinch at the wrist), shoulder tendonitis (biceps, rotator cuff), thoracic outlet syndrome (pinched nerve at the shoulder), and / or neck strain, neck herniated disk, pinched nerve, and/or headaches. Many times, these conditions co-exist if the patient has really abused themselves (such as music majors who may practice playing their instrument for 4-5 hours a day) to a point where they are REALLY injured in multiple areas.

Limiting this discussion to pinched nerves in the neck and upper limb, the question often arises, "…how do you know where the nerve is pinched?" The answer centers around determining an accurate history to find out EXACTLY where the patient feels numbness, tingling, weakness, and/or pain as each nerve innervates a different area. For example, if a patient says, "…I feel numbness in my 4th and 5th finger," this tells us that the ulnar nerve is pinched (as opposed to numbness in the 2nd, 3rd, or 4th fingers which suggests median nerve pinch—more classic of CTS). If the patient says the numbness affects the arm from the elbow down to the 4th and 5th finger, this suggests cubital tunnel syndrome (ulnar nerve pinch at the medial elbow). If the numbness affects the person from the shoulder to the 4th and 5th finger, thoracic outlet syndrome becomes a probable diagnosis. And lastly, if the neck, shoulder, arm and hand on the pinky side are numb, we are suspicious of a pinched nerve in the neck.

Then, we confirm our suspicions with a more detailed physical examination. Here, we test for compression of a nerve at the neck by positioning the head in a backwards, rotated position and holding it for about 10 seconds to see if the numbness is reproduced. We can also manually (with our hands/fingers) compress the various nerve pathways to see if numbness occurs at the front of the neck, the shoulder under the collar bone, at the elbow and wrist counting the seconds to time the onset of numbness and mapping the numbness location. Placing the shoulder, elbow, and wrist in different positions can pinch the nerve as well, and mapping the location of the numbness tells us where and to what degree the nerve is pinched. We will also perform a neurological exam testing reflexes and strength, as well as sensory function using a sharp object. A special test called an EMG/NCV (electromyography and nerve conduction velocity) can be obtained to further verify the location and degree of nerve pinching and damage.

The advantage of chiropractic management is that we will treat EVERY LOCATION that may be contributing to the CTS symptoms, whether the pinch is in the neck, shoulder, elbow and/or wrist. Managing the WHOLE PERSON, not just the wrist or CTS is KEY to a successful outcome.

Carpal Tunnel Syndrome – What Makes My Hands Numb?

Carpal Tunnel Syndrome (CTS) sufferers frequently report a cluster of symptoms, but almost all have one symptom in common – numbness, usually in digits 2-4 on palm-side of the hand. CTS is usually attributed to an over-use type of injury such as repetitive work including (but not limited to): typing, assembly work, packaging jobs, machine operators, and many more. Last month, we discussed CTS "Facts" and learned many important points about CTS. This month's focus centers around the common question, "....where is this numbness coming from?"

To answer this, let's review the anatomy: The carpal tunnel is made up of 8 small "carpal bones" that form an arch or tunnel, and the base of the tunnel is formed from the transverse carpal ligament. There are nine tendons that attach muscles in the forearm to each finger and work when we grip or form a fist with our hand. Wiggle your fingers and look at your wrist and forearm – do you see all the activity or movement going on?

The tendons travel through sheaths which help lubricate the sliding tendons. When we move our fingers fast (such as typing, playing piano, performing assembly work, etc.), friction and heat builds up, resulting in swelling. If adequate rest does not occur, the increased pressure from the swollen tendons end up squeezing all the contents within the tunnel, which includes the median nerve. It's the median nerve pinch that results in the numbness, tingling, and/or pain into the index, third and forth fingers.

There are other conditions that can either complicate or cause CTS. These include: hypothyroid disease (due to myxedema), diabetes (due to neuropathy), inflammatory arthritis (of which there are several kinds - rheumatoid is the most common), and pinching of the nerve either in the neck, shoulder, elbow or forearm (called double or multiple crush syndrome).

The reason chiropractic helps so much is that we can alleviate the pressure on the nerve from the neck down to the wrist and restore nerve function. This alleviates the multiple sleep interruptions, weakness in the grip that is so common, as well as helping to restore the nerve's function. Many studies support the success of chiropractic and CTS – try it first as surgery should be the last resort.

Carpal Tunnel Syndrome – 13 Fun Facts!

Carpal Tunnel Syndrome (CTS) results in numbness, tingling, and sometimes weak grip strength due pinching of the median nerve as it travels through the carpal tunnel at the wrist. There are many conditions that are similar to CTS, many of which we have discussed in the past. The following is a list of "13 fun facts" aimed at helping to properly identify CTS, knowing what to do about it, and at helping to make an informed decision as to whom to seek help for it.

1. CTS is most common in women, age >50, who work in a repetitive, rapid moving manually demanding occupation (typing/computer work, line assembly work, waiting tables, and more).
2. CTS is complicated by the presence of obesity, diabetes, hypothyroid, pregnancy, taking birth control pills, and other conditions that cause inflammation (rheumatoid arthritis and others).
3. CTS may develop on the dominant side, the non-dominant side or both—each case is individual.

4. CTS symptoms may FIRST present as morning or night time numbness that can wake the sufferer up once or many times during the night.
5. CTS sufferers USUALLY wait for weeks, months or even years before seeking help for it, which is a risk factor for a delayed recovery – GET HELP ASAP!!!
6. CTS can often be managed without surgery—especially IF you have it treated sooner rather than later.
7. CTS surgery may be necessary if non-surgical care fails. This may be due to the nerve being damaged beyond a certain point (an EMG/NCV or, electromyography/nerve conduction velocity helps determine this along with an accurate history and examination).
8. CTS non-surgical care includes: chiropractic manipulation of the wrist, elbow, shoulder and/or neck—depending on the case. All health care providers usually include a night wrist splint, anti-inflammatory measures, ergonomic modifications of work stations, and stretching exercises.
9. CTS non-surgical success favors chiropractic because of the inclusion of the manual therapies. When only exercise, night splinting, and NSAIDS are used, the success rate drops off dramatically.
10. Reduced thyroid function makes CTS worse because of the unique type of swelling associated with hypothyroidism called "myxedema." Because of the confined space available in the carpal tunnel, a small amount of swelling can result in nerve compression and the classic numbness/tingling symptoms in the middle three fingers on the palm-side of the hand.
11. CTS is worse at night because it is impossible to control the position of the wrist while we sleep. As a result, we tend to curl the wrist and hand under our chin, and when the wrist bends forwards or backwards, the pressure inside the carpal tunnel increases significantly due to the change in tunnel size. This is why wearing a wrist splint at night REALLY HELPS as it keeps the wrist from bending, keeping the tunnel as wide as possible, thus lowering the pressure within it.
12. CTS patients respond well in some cases to vitamin B6. This is due to the healing effects of B6 (peridoxine) on neuropathy and/or it's anti-inflammatory qualities. Other anti-inflammatory nutrients include ginger, turmeric,

boswellia, bioflavinoids, white willow bark, quercetin, and others.

13. CTS patients do not always improve after surgery. This can be due to the fact that the median nerve is frequently "pinched" in more than one area such as the neck, thoracic outlet (shoulder), pronator tunnel (elbow) as well as at the wrist. When more than one compression is present, this is referred to as "double" or "multiple crush syndrome."

Carpal Tunnel Syndrome – Are There Other Tunnels?

Carpal Tunnel Syndrome (CTS) refers to the median nerve being pinched in a tunnel at the wrist. As the name implies, "carpal" refers to the 8 small bones in the wrist that make up the "U" shaped part of the tunnel and "syndrome" means symptoms that are specific and unique to this condition. As we learned last month, CTS can be affected by nerve pinches more proximal to the wrist, such as at the forearm, elbow, mid-upper arm, shoulder or neck. To make matters more complex, there are two other nerves in the arm that can also be pinched in different tunnels, and the symptoms of numbing and tingling in the arm and hand occur with those conditions as well. This is why a careful clinical history, examination, and sometimes special tests like an EMG/NCV (electromyogram/nerve conduction velocity) offer the information that allows for an accurate diagnosis of one or more of these "tunnel syndromes" in the "CTS" patient. Let's look at these different tunnels and their associated symptoms, as this will help you understand the ways we can differentiate between these various syndromes or conditions.

Let's start at the neck . There are seven cervical vertebrae and eight cervical spinal nerves that exit the spine through a small hole called the IVF (intervertebral foramen). Each nerve, like a wire to a light, goes specifically to a known location which includes: the head (nerves C1, 2, 3), the neck and shoulders (C4, 5), the thumb side of the arm (C6), the middle hand and finger (C7) and the pinky side of the lower arm and hand (C8). If a nerve gets pinched at the spinal level (such as a herniated disk in the neck), usually there is numbness, tingling, and/or pain and sometimes, usually a little later, weakness in the affected part/s of the arm and hand (or numbness in the scalp if it's a C1-3 nerve pinch). So, we as chiropractors can test the patient's sensation using light touch, pin prick, vibration, and/or 2-points brought progressively closer together until 1-point is perceived and then comparing it to the other arm/hand. Reflexes and muscle strength are also tested to see if the motor part of the nerve is involved in the pinch. The exam includes compression tests of the neck to see if the arm "lights up" with symptoms during the test.

Next is the shoulder . Here, the nerves and blood vessels travel through an opening between the collar bone, 1st rib and the chest muscles (Pectorals). As you might think, the nerves and blood vessels can be stretched and pinched as they travel through this opening and can cause "thoracic outlet syndrome." Symptoms occur when we raise the arm overhead. Hence, our tests include checking the pulse at the wrist to see if it reduces or lessens in intensity as we raise the arm over the head. At the shoulder, the ulnar nerve is the most commonly pinched nerve, which will make the pinky side of the arm and hand numb, tingly, and/or painful. A less common place to pinch the nerves is along humerus bone (upper arm) by a bony process and ligament that is usually not there or resulting from a fracture. Here, an x-ray will show the problem.

The elbow is the MOST common place to trap the ulnar nerve in the "cubital tunnel" located at the inner elbow near the "funny bone" which we have all bumped more than once. Cubital tunnel syndrome affects the pinky side of the hand from the elbow down. The median/carpal tunnel nerve can get trapped here by the pronator teres muscle, thus "pronator tunnel syndrome." This COMMONLY accompanies CTS and MUST be treated to obtain good results with CTS patients. The radial nerve can be trapped at the radial tunnel located on the outside of the elbow and creates thumb side and back of the hand numbness/tingling.

Hence, you see the importance of evaluating and treating ALL the tunnels when CTS is present so a thorough job is done (which is what Chiropractors do). Try the LEAST invasive approach first – non-surgical treatment – as it's usually all that is needed!

CTS - MD vs. DC. Whom Should I See?

Carpal Tunnel Syndrome (CTS) is a very common problem affecting a large population (1 out of 20 in the general population) including typists, assembly line workers, postal employees, secretaries, servers/waiters, musicians, carpenters, and many others. CTS drives a high level of cost to the health care system between time lost from work, treatment costs, and short and long term disability payments (on average $30,000 per claim, and this is an old stat!). Continued CTS signs and symptoms can persist long after surgical treatment and the question that typically arises when this happens is "…why?" Let's take a look at reasons for failed treatment of CTS…

The classic non-surgical medical management model for treating CTS includes non-steroidal, anti-inflammatory medication (like ibuprofen), rest, and the use of nocturnal (night time) wrist splints. This approach works in some cases, but in the majority, it is unsuccessful and leads to the next medical management step: surgery.

The classic chiropractic management model for treating CTS includes similar initial treatment approaches including anti-inflammatory measures, rest, and night wrist splints. One anti-inflammatory measure is ice massage or cupping, where the ice is rubbed directly on the skin until numbness is achieved (this usually takes about 4 minutes). Prior to numbness, there will be a burning and aching often described as intense, "…like a brain-freeze when I drink a slushy too fast." The ice cup approach can be repeated several times a day. Other anti-inflammatory measures may include the use of herbal anti-inflammatory nutrients such as ginger, tumeric, boswellia, bioflavinoids, and/or the use of digestive enzymes taken between meals to help reduce the inflammation. The "rest" component is also shared by both models as is the use of the night wrist splint. So, what makes the chiropractic model different?

The nerve affected in CTS is called the median nerve. It arises initially from the nerves in the neck, specifically, C6-8 and T1 nerve roots which are part of the brachial plexus. These form into one nerve (the median nerve) which travels through small openings, first at the neck followed by the shoulder (called the thoracic outlet), then into the arm through a muscle at the elbow (pronator tunnel), and finally through the carpal tunnel at the wrist to innervate the hand including the palm and the 2nd, 3rd digits and thumb side of the 4th finger. The median nerve can get "crushed" in more than one tunnel and treatment must address the WHOLE nerve, not just at the carpal tunnel / wrist. This chiropractic management of CTS helps many patients because the nerve along its entire course including the neck, shoulder, and elbow is treated, not just the wrist!

Carpal Tunnel Syndrome and Self-Help Management Options

Carpal Tunnel Syndrome (CTS) is the most investigated, researched, and talked about disorder when it comes to work related injuries to the upper extremity because it is often the cause of so much lost work time, disability costs, and the source of financial hardship for many of its sufferers. So, the questions are: Is there a way to detect it early? What can be done to prevent CTS? And, what can you do to facilitate in the treatment process of CTS?

1. EARLY DETECTION: Because CTS symptoms usually start out mildly, maybe a little numbness or tingling in the hand or fingers that can be easily "shaken off," people usually do not identify these early symptoms as, "...a big

deal" and consequently, do nothing about it. After a while, and the time depends on how severely the median nerve is pinched, you may start waking up at night needing to shake out your hands in order to return to sleep. Similarly, when driving, you may need to change your hand position on the steering wheel due to the same symptoms. If you are really stubborn (and many people are) and you STILL don't give in and come to us for treatment, then buttoning shirts, writing, crocheting, knitting, playing piano, typing, etc., may all soon become affected. The KEY in early detection is to NOT ignore the early symptoms. Come in right away!

2. PREVENTION: There are many highly effective preventative tactics. For example, recognize that certain conditions predispose us to CTS and anything to avoid and/or properly manage these conditions will help. Some of these conditions include diabetes mellitus, pregnancy, the use of birth control pills, inflammatory arthritis (such as rheumatoid or lupus), hypothyroidism, and obesity. From an ergonomic approach, make sure your work station is set up properly including (but not limited to) the position of the monitor, the keyboard, the mouse, and your chair. Set up the area so the extremes of wrist bending can be avoided. If a wrist brace doesn't get in the way, it may help, especially when there is a high incidence rate of CTS with your co-workers. Most importantly, small mini-breaks and stretching can be highly effective during the day. If you develop any symptoms, come in and see us RIGHT AWAY (see #1 above).

3. SELF-MANAGEMENT: Certainly consider and implement the "prevention" approaches described above in #2. Specific exercises for stretching, strengthening, and dexterity REALLY HELP! We will teach you these, as it is important that you perform the correct exercises accurately. Improper exercising will only add to the problems that lead to CTS or, worsen it. Control your diet to avoid obesity, to control diabetes and the other sometimes preventable conditions described above. Wearing a wrist splint, especially at night can also really help. There are many types from Velcro wrist wraps with or without thumb loops to cock-up splints, carpal lock splints, and many more. The key as to whether to use a

wrist splint or not during work is largely dependent on the comfort of the splint during the work day. Many occupations simply require too much wrist bending or movement for the splint to be comfortably worn during the work day which ends up bruising the forearm and/or hand due to the repetitive motion into the edges of the splint. If or when daytime use of the splint isn't tolerated, use it only at night to prevent extreme wrist bending while sleeping. This usually REALLY helps. Bottom line, remember the saying, "…an ounce of prevention is worth a pound of cure!"

CTS – Natural Treatment Options

Carpal Tunnel Syndrome (CTS) is a condition characterized by pain, numbness and/or tingling in the hand. This includes the palm and the 2nd, 3rd, and half of the 4th finger, usually sparing the thumb. Another indication of CTS is weakness in grip strength such as difficulty opening a jar to even holding a coffee cup. CTS can occur from many different causes, the most common being repetitive motion injuries such as assembly line or typing/computing work. Here is a PARTIAL list of potential causes of CTS: heredity (a small sized tunnel), aging (>50 years old), rheumatoid arthritis, pregnancy, hypothyroid, birth control pill use, trauma to the wrist (especially colles fractures), diabetes mellitus, acromegaly, the use of corticosteroids, tumors (benign or malignant), obesity (BMI>29 are 2.5 more likely), double crush (pinching of the nerve in more than 1 place such as the neck and the carpal tunnel), heterozygous mutations in a gene (associated with Charcot-Marie-Tooth), Parvovirus b19, and others. Again, repetitive trauma is still the most common cause. It becomes quite clear that a COMPLETE physical examination must be conducted, not just evaluation of the wrist! Once the cause(s) of CTS has been nailed down, then treatment options can be considered.

From a treatment perspective, we've previously discussed what chiropractors typically do for CTS (spinal and extremity joint manipulation, muscle/soft tissue mobilization, physical therapy modalities such as laser, the use of a wrist splint – especially at night, work task modifications, wrist/hand/arm/neck exercises, vitamin B6, and more). But, what about using other "alternative" or non-medical approaches, especially those that can be done with chiropractic treatment? Here is a list of four alternative or complementary treatment options:

1. Anti-inflammatory Goals: Reducing systemic inflammation reduces overall pressure on the median nerve that travels through the limited space within the carpal tunnel at the wrist. An "anti-inflammatory diet" such a Mediterranean diet, gluten-free diet, paleo-diet (also referred to as the caveman diet) can also help. Herbs that can helps include arnica, bromelain, white willow bark, curcumen, ginger, turmeric, boswellia, and vitamins such as bioflavinoids, Vitamin B6 (and other B vitamins such as B1 and B12), vitamin C, and also omega 3 fatty acids.
2. Acupuncture: Inserting very thin needles into specific acupuncture points both near the wrist and further away can unblock energy channels (called meridians), improve energy flow, release natural pain reducing chemicals (endorphins and enkephlins), promote circulation and balance the nervous system. For CTS, the acupuncture points are located on the wrist, arm, thumb, hand, neck, upper back and leg. The number of sessions varies, dependant on how long the CTS has been present, the person's overall health, and the severity of CTS.
3. Laser acupuncture: The use of a low level (or "cold" laser) or a class IV pulsed laser over the same acupuncture points as mentioned above can have very similar beneficial effects (without needles)! One particular study of 36 subjects with CTS for an average of 24 months included 14 patients who had 1-2 prior surgeries for CTS with poor post-surgical results. Even in that group, improvement was reported after 3 laser treatments per week for 4-5 weeks! In total, 33 of the 36 subjects reported 50-100% relief. These benefits were reportedly long-term as follow-up at 1-2 years later showed only 2 out of 23 subjects had pain that returned

and subsequent laser treatment was again successful within several weeks.

4. Acupressure: Acupuncture point stimulation with manual pressure. These points can be self-stimulated by the CTS sufferer multiple times a day via deep rubbing techniques.

Carpal Tunnel Syndrome – Prevention Tactics

Carpal Tunnel Syndrome (CTS) is a very common problem that is often associated with work-related activities. This article focuses on how to prevent CTS. Of course, if you already have CTS, you should still read this in order to learn preventative measures that also work while you receive treatment for your condition.

The concept is to think about prevention as a matter of economics. As you lose time from work because of CTS, if affects your bottom line, and I'm sure you have bills to pay and mouths to feed (…or at least one)! So please take the advice offered here seriously, as we are genuine about our concern for your well-being and not losing work time is a huge component of all of our "well-being!"

If you've experienced sore wrists or hands, sudden sharp jabs of pain up the forearm, noted numbness and/or burning in your fingers (especially the index through 4th / ring finger), wake up at night needing to shake and flick your fingers to "wake them up," have weakness in your grip strength, are slowing down at work (whether it's typing/computer work, assembly line work, cooking, serving tables, and so on), then you likely NEED to do the following NOW! The goal here is prevent work loss and surgery (as up to six weeks of lost work time will be required if surgery is needed).

1. Anti-inflammatory measures: This starts with a healthy diet. STOP eating foods that inflame such as omega-6 fatty acid-rich foods ("GOOGLE" omega-6 and print out

the list of food). Emphasize fruits, vegetables, lean meats, and nuts and AVOID grains because of glutens, which many of us have a sensitivity against. Vitamins such as a multiple, magnesium, fish oil (omega 3 fatty acids), vitamin D3, and CoQ10 are GREAT! Freeze water in a small cup and rub it on the wrist/carpal tunnel until it gets numb (takes 3-5 minutes) and do that 2-3 times a day. Consider natural anti-inflammatories such as ginger, turmeric, cercumen, bioflavinoides, and others.

2. Stretch: Bear-claw, fist, "High-5" (opened hand with the fingers fanned out) reps, wrist extensions on the wall/table stretches (elbows straight).

3. Rest: Cock-up splint, take mini-breaks, and get sound/restoring sleep. IT REALLY HELPS!

4. Ergonomic modifications: Position your computer keyboard, mouse and monitor so that you are looking straight ahead at a slight downward angle and your elbows are at a 90° or slightly less of an angle when typing. Set an alarm on your computer to go off every 15 minutes as a reminder to "shake and flick" your hands, wiggle your fingers, do your stretches, and/or squeeze a soft ball. Write with a fat pen vs. a skinny one – this helps a lot!

5. Weight management: Obesity is a common risk factor for developing CTS.

6. Manage other health issues: Diabetes, thyroid disease, inflammatory arthritis, neck/shoulder or elbow problems can all contribute to or even cause CTS.

Think of the above measures as minimums and obtain professional care to help you further. You have choices between the traditional medical model of cortisone shots, anti-inflammatory medication, and surgery vs. chiropractic care which includes manipulation and mobilization of the fingers, hand, wrist, elbow, shoulder, and neck as needed, splinting at night, anti-inflammatory diet and nutrients, ergonomic modification, and exercise training, which ALL will help to treat as well as prevent future CTS problems, EVEN IF you've had surgery already!

Carpal Tunnel Syndrome – A Yoga Class!

Carpal Tunnel Syndrome (CTS) is a very common problem that affects many people. In fact, the US Bureau of Labor Statistics reports about 28,000 CTS cases per year and because so many sufferers jump to a surgical option, it's become THE LEADING CAUSE of lost workdays in the United States. Women are 71% more likely more likely to develop CTS than men!

In a review of over 31,000 cases, women spent an average of 30 days off work because of CTS. Jobs most commonly affected include: production workers in food processing and clothing manufacturing, typists who work at keyboards for hours on end, and construction workers who use tools that vibrate, such as jackhammers or tools that have poorly designed handles. The Journal of the American Medical Association recently estimated that almost 3 percent of adults in the United States may suffer from Carpal Tunnel Syndrome at some point in their lives.

Now that we've learned how susceptible we are to CTS, what are some things you can do to decrease your chances of acquiring Carpal Tunnel Syndrome? For starters, keep your weight reasonable (Body Mass Index between 19 and 25), take "mini-breaks" during the repetitive work day, and receive chiropractic treatments aimed at releasing the tight muscles in the neck, shoulders, upper arms, forearms, hand and adjusting the associated joints.

You can also stretch! There are many different types of stretches that should be considered. Feel free to watch the entire 37-minute YouTube video at the link below that addresses many exercises that may help:
As you perform these various stretches, take deep breaths, "feel" the different fibers of muscles stretch and keep the intensity, "…within reasonable pain boundaries." That is, a "good hurt" is what you're striving for here, no sharp pain is allowed!

Carpal Tunnel Syndrome and Vitamin B6

Carpal Tunnel Syndrome (CTS) is a common condition usually associated with repetitive strain from jobs that require a fast, constant movement of the arms and hands (such as working on an assembly line). Up to 9% of adult women develop CTS and the incidence increases after age 50. A common medical treatment approach has been a combination of drugs (including corticosteroids), diuretics, splinting at night, and modifying activities, often including a "light duty" status until the symptoms calm down. Prior to accepting surgery as, "…the only option left," an "alternative treatment" approach of vitamin B6 (and of course, chiropractic manual therapies) is chosen by many. Many treatment approaches have been previously discussed; however, today, we'll take a closer look at the vitamin B6 /CTS connection.

Research regarding the use of vitamin B6 or, pyridoxine, can be traced way back into the '70s and '80s when it was reported that B6 is involved in several metabolic pathways, including neural function ("neurotransmission"). This is how it helps CTS patients since CTS occurs as the consequence of a pinched (median) nerve at the wrist. Findings from the initial studies, though quite small in terms of the number of subjects, suggested B6 improved the symptoms of CTS (such as, numbness and tingling into the 2nd to 4th palm-side fingers) by raising the pain threshold (that is, the point when symptoms occurred). Another study reported improvements in pain scores and mild improvements in electromyography and nerve conduction velocity (EMG-NCV) studies. Another study reported that at least 7 patients in their study were B6 deficient when blood tested. Regarding the dose, one study reported that taking only 2mg of B6 was enough to improve the patient's CTS symptoms, but 100mg was needed for the avoidance of surgery. In a large "retrospective literature review" of 994 CTS patient files, it was reported that when 494 patients were treated with 100mg twice a day, the rate of symptom alleviation was 68%, much higher than group that did not receive B6 (only 14.3%). Yet, controversy is still reported about the effectiveness of B6 and firm conclusions are lacking. Despite this uncertainty, 200 mg of vitamin B6 is frequently included as part of the non-surgical "package" (along with NSAIDs like ibuprofen, nighttime splints, and an ergonomic workstation evaluation).

So, how much B6 is "enough?" The recommended daily intake is only 2 mg or less for all ages, genders and lifestyles with an upper limit set at 100 mg/day. The main toxicity issue is sensory neuropathy, which (oddly) is very similar to the symptoms caused by CTS! The good news is that CTS symptoms rapidly disappear at doses < 1000 mg/day and most studies indicate no toxic neuropathy by taking doses between 40 and 500 mg/day. Hence, it is recommended to never exceed 500mg/day and most recommendations are in the 100-200 mg/day range. If symptoms improve, a gradual reduction in the dose after about 3 months is advised. Closer monitoring of symptoms in those taking >200mg/day is recommended, especially since the symptoms of toxicity and CTS are so similar. Other B6 toxicity symptoms include depression, fatigue, impaired memory, irritability, headaches, altered walking, and bloating. So, keep your eyes open if doses >200mg/day are taken. Other micronutrients to consider that are anti-inflammatory in nature include omega 3 fatty acids, vitamin D, magnesium (often in combination with calcium), Co-Q10, proteolytic enzymes, and herbs such as ginger, tumeric, boswellia, white willow bark and more.

Carpal Tunnel Syndrome Management

In many cases, Carpal Tunnel Syndrome (CTS) results strictly from overuse activities though, as we have discussed previously, other conditions such as hypothyroid, taking birth control pills, pregnancy, diabetes, obesity, certain types of arthritis, etc. can also be involved as a contributor and / or the sole cause. When these conditions are present, they must be properly treated to achieve a favorable result. However, the majority of cases are the result of a repetitive motion injury. So, the question remains:

What is the role of the patient regarding activity modification during the treatment process of CTS? How important is it?

To answer this question, let's look at a fairly common type of CTS case. In our hypothetical case, the patient is female, 52 years old, moderately obese (Body Mass Index 35 where the normal is 19-25), and works for a local cookie packing company. Her job is to stand on a line where cookies are traveling down a conveyor belt after being baked and cooled. She reaches forwards with both arms and grasps the cookies, sometimes several at a time, and places them into plastic packaging which are then wrapped and finally removed from the belt and placed into boxes located at the end of the line. Each worker rotates positions every 30 minutes. A problem can occur when other workers fall behind or when there aren't enough workers on the line, at which time the speed required to complete the job increases.

So now, let's discuss the "pathology" behind CTS. The cause of CTS is the pinching of the median nerve inside the carpal tunnel, located on the palm side of the wrist. The tunnel is made up of 2 rows of 4 carpal bones that form top of the tunnel while a ligament stretches across, making up the tunnel's floor. There are 9 tendons that travel through the tunnel and "during rush hour" (or, when the worker is REALLY moving fast, trying to keep up with production), the friction created between the tendons, their sheaths (covering) and surrounding synovial lining (a lubricating membrane that covers the tendons sheaths), results in inflammation or swelling. When this happens, there just isn't enough room inside the tunnel for the additional swelling and everything gets compressed. The inflamed contents inside the tunnel push the median nerve (that also travels through the tunnel) against the ligament and pinched nerve symptoms occur (numbness, tingling, and loss of the grip strength). The worker notices significant problems at night when her hands interrupt her sleep and she has to shake and flick her fingers to try to get them to "wake up." She notices that only the index to the 3rd and thumb half of the 4th finger are numb, primarily on the palm side.

At this stage, the worker often waits to see if this is just a temporary problem that will go away on its own and if not, she'll make an appointment for a consultation, often at her family doctor (since many patients don't realize chiropractic treatments REALLY HELP this condition). In an "ideal world," the primary care doctor first refers the patient to the chiropractor for non-surgical management. Other treatment elements include the use of a night wrist splint, ice massage over the tunnel, and possibly modality treatments such as low level laser therapy and (one of the MOST IMPORTANT) "ergonomic management." That means work station modifications, which may include slowing down the line, the addition 1 or 2 workers, and reducing the reach requirement by adding a "rake" that pushes the cookies towards the worker/s. Strict home instructions to allow for proper rest and managing home repetitive tasks are also very important. Between all these approaches, chiropractic is HIGHLY SUCCESSFUL in managing the CTS patient, but it may require a workstation analysis.

Carpal Tunnel Syndrome and Chiropractic

Carpal Tunnel Syndrome (CTS) is a very common problem. The American Association of Orthopedic Surgeons (AAOS) reported that in 2007, there were 330,000 carpal tunnel release surgeries performed. The main reason to have the surgery is to "open up" the tunnel. That is, the transverse carpal ligament or "floor" of the tunnel is released so the contents inside the tunnel are able to move more freely, reducing the pressure inside the tunnel. Essentially, this is the goal of any treatment (surgical or not): improving the depth of the tunnel, thus reducing the pressure from inside the tunnel allowing the tendons to slide better as the muscles on the palm-side forearm contract to move the nine tendons that pass through the tunnel and attach to the fingers and thumb. However, there are non-surgical methods for reducing the pressure within the tunnel that should be first attempted as surgery is always reported to be the "...last resort" for good reason. There can be surgical complications, the effects may be only partial, and there is an average of 30% grip strength loss following the transverse ligament surgical release. So, the question is, how can chiropractic approaches reduce the pressure inside the carpal tunnel without somehow changing the length of the transverse carpal ligament?

The roof of the tunnel is made up of two rows of four bones for a total of eight carpal bones that arch over the nine tendons that pass through the tunnel. The height of the tunnel is dependant on the position of those eight bones, especially three of the eight bones that make up the proximal row at the top of the cave. These are technically the lunate (located at the peak of the roof which tends to drop down lowering the roof of the tunnel), the scaphoid (located on the thumb side of the roof), and the triquetrum (located on the pinky side of the roof). The latter two bones tend to shift up and out and when the middle bone drops down, the tunnel flattens making the space tighter or smaller. This is how chiropractic adjustments of the wrist help. There are specific techniques we use to reposition the lunate and outer two bones that shift up and out. In addition, we can either tape or use an elastic wristband to hold the tunnel "open" after the adjustment.

The use of a night splint to keep the wrist in a straight or slightly "cocked-up" position is also highly beneficial as the pressure inside the tunnel goes up as much as 6-8x when CTS is present when the wrist bends to the end points of upward or downward bending. Also, we will treat all the possible points of possible compression including the neck, shoulder, elbow, forearm and wrist which ALWAYS gets better results than treating only the carpal tunnel.

Carpal Tunnel Syndrome: 3 Great Exercises!

Because carpal tunnel syndrome (CTS) is technically a tendonitis that happens to be near a nerve (the median nerve), one treatment option for CTS is to manage the tendonitis and by doing so, the pressure on the median nerve will resolve. Also, because the movement of the hand and wrist are controlled by opposite functioning muscles (that is, when we flex the wrist and fingers, the palm side tendons are doing the job and when we extend the wrist/fingers, the back of the forearm and hand tendons are doing the work), these opposite functioning actions need to be balanced. Moreover, if the muscles on one side of the forearm are tight and inflamed, very often so are the muscles on the opposite side.

Therefore, an exercise program for the forearm and hand should include BOTH sides, not just the flexor or palm side of the forearm/hand where the carpal tunnel is located. Perform these exercises multiple times a day for 3-10 second hold times. You can modify #2 and #3 by NOT using the opposite hand to pull but rather, simply make the movement without the opposite hand assisting in the stretch. That way, you can perform BOTH at the same time IF your time is short (such as when performing these during a busy work day, for example).

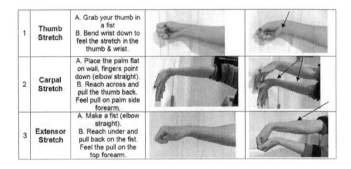

1	Thumb Stretch	A. Grab your thumb in a fist B. Bend wrist down to feel the stretch in the thumb & wrist.		
2	Carpal Stretch	A. Place the palm flat on wall, fingers point down (elbow straight). B. Reach across and pull the thumb back. Feel pull on palm side forearm.		
3	Extensor Stretch	A. Make a fist (elbow straight). B. Reach under and pull back on the fist. Feel the pull on the top forearm.		

Feel for the stretch where the arrows are pointing – it should be a "good" hurt/stretch!

Carpal Tunnel Syndrome: Prevention

People who spend a lot of time performing activities that require a high level of force, repetition, or use vibrating tools are at risk of developing carpal tunnel syndrome (CTS). Other activities such as driving, playing musical instruments, knitting, using a sander, screw drivers, air wrenches, waitress work, or assembling small parts are also associated with increased CTS risk. The good news: there are ways we can reduce the risk of developing CTS. Some of these include the following:

1. Stay Healthy: There are many conditions that contribute to the onset and/or make CTS worse. Exercise, maintain a healthy weight (Body Mass Index – BMI – of 25 or less), stop smoking (or better yet, never start), take your thyroid medication (if indicated), keep your blood sugar normal (obesity leads to diabetes which often worsens CTS), and do your carpal tunnel exercises multiple times a day.
2. Ergonomics: Use "ergonomic" principles when arranging your workstation such as sitting properly at your home and work computers. The placement of your desk, the computer monitor, the keyboard (consider a convex keyboard rather than the flat type), the mouse (and type of mouse – the track ball mouse requires no arm movement, only the thumb), paperwork space and location. The type of chair and its height are also very important. Avoid desks that have sharp edges as they can compress the forearms and pinch the CTS nerve.
3. Posture: The position in which you sit is important! Sit in an upright position, head/chin tucked in, feet on the floor or on a box, elbows resting on adjustable arms of the chair bent about 90 degrees, and keep your wrists fairly straight/neutral. Avoid slouching, reaching out with the elbows less than 90 degrees, head shifted forwards and shoulders rounded and feet not positioned under you. When you talk on the phone, STRONGLY consider a headset! Pinching the phone between your shoulder and ear with your head bent sideways for any length of time is a ticket to disaster for developing CTS and/or other types of cumulative trauma disorders (pinched nerves in

the neck, shoulder tendonitis/bursitis, elbow tendonitis and more).

4. Plan your activities: Pay careful attention to your daily routine for activities that may increase your risk of developing or perpetuating CTS. For example, these activities can increase your chance of developing or worsening CTS: playing a musical instrument, knitting, carpentry, playing video or computer games for hours, working on cars, operating vibrating tools, using forceful gripping such as spray bottles, using a crutch, cane, wheelchair, engaging in certain sports such as long-distance cycling that load the arm and hand, skiing – waterskiing requires a firm grip on the handle and snow skiing requires firm gripping on the ski pole.

5. Sleep: It is impossible to control the position we put our hands/wrists in at night. Therefore, it is essential to wear wrist splints so we avoid bending the wrists in our sleep. Many of us curl up in a ball and tuck or bend the wrists and hands under our chin. In a "normal" wrist, the pressure inside the carpal tunnel DOUBLES when we bend our wrists! If we have CTS, the pressure goes up exponentially or, 6-8 times because of the increased pressure that's there already because of the CTS. Use a pillow that is designed for you, we'll help you with that!

6. Take a break! It's important to pace yourself if your work or play includes fast, repetitive activities. It's easy to get lost into what you're doing so a timer to remind you that an hour has gone by and to take a break is a wise purchase. There are computer programs that flash on your screen, "Time to stretch!" Some of these may include the actual exercise so you don't forget what to do. If not, talk to us about what exercises are good to do either at the workstation and/or at home for CTS.

Carpal Tunnel Syndrome and Sleeping

Have you ever woken up in the middle of the night and noticed your hand sleeping to the point where you had to get out of bed and shake or flick your fingers to alleviate the numbness? If the numbness was primarily on the thumb-side half of your hand, it may have been carpal tunnel syndrome that woke you up. So, the question is, why is it such an issue at night?

To properly answer this question, let's get familiar with the anatomy of the wrist. There are 2 bones that make up the forearm – the ulna (on the pinky side) and the radius (on the thumb side). Just beyond that, there are two rows of four bones each called the carpal bones for a total of 8 small bones that make up the wrist joint. These carpal bones are arranged in a horseshoe or tunnel shape. When you look down at your wrist and wiggle your fingers quickly, you can see all the movement that occurs on the palm side of the wrist. That's a lot of movement! You can also see the muscles on the upper half of the forearm moving rapidly as the fingers wiggle.

There are 9 muscle tendons that travel through the carpal tunnel, as well as some blood vessels and most important, the median nerve sits on top of all those moving tendons. Just beneath the floor of the tunnel is a ligament called the transverse carpal ligament. The tendons inside the tunnel are surrounded by lubricating sheaths that make it easier for the tendons to slide back and forth as we wiggle our fingers, grip to open a jar, type on a computer, play a musical instrument, or so on. Without the tendon sheaths, the friction between the rubbing tendons would quickly build up heat, resulting in swelling, pain and numbness. However, in spite of the lubricating function of the sheaths, when we work our fingers and hands too much, swelling and inflammation does occur.

So, why do we have numbness at night when we aren't working, gripping and moving our fingers repetitively? The answer lies in how we sleep. Since we are asleep, we cannot control where we position our hands and wrists. Most of us curl up in a ball and tuck our hands under our chin or someplace cozy. Normally, when we bend our wrists, the pressure inside the carpal tunnel doubles. However, a carpal tunnel patient already has a higher level of pressure in their wrist. So, when a carpal tunnel patient bends their wrist in the exact same way, the pressure goes up even more – that is, 3, 4, 5, or more times than a normal person without their wrist bent. That is why a wrist "cock-up" splint works so well at night! It keeps the wrist straight so we can't bend it. Often, this allows the CTS patient to sleep through the night instead of waking up 2, 3, or more times with numbness, tingling, and/or pain on the thumb half of the hand.

CTS – Why Braces Work

When patients present for treatment of carpal tunnel syndrome (CTS), one of the most common treatments rendered is the use of a wrist brace, often referred to as a cock-up splint. The focus of this article is to explain the reasons why these braces are so commonly included in the management of CTS and why they work.

CTS is caused by anything that applies pressure on the median nerve (see #9 in C, D & E below) in a tight space called the carpal tunnel (see A & B below). The tunnel is made up of 8 bones that form the "U" shaped part of the tunnel while the floor or bottom of the tunnel is made up of a ligament called the transverse carpal ligament. There are also 9 tendons (tendons are structures that attach muscles to bones) and their coverings or sheaths that are needed to reduce friction as the tendons slide back and forth, such as when our fingers type on a computer, open the lid of a jar, lift a suitcase, hold a pen or pencil when writing, open a door knob, button a shirt... the list goes on and on! If the tendons didn't have a sheath to slide in, the friction would build up too quickly, causing swelling and pain from tendonitis. The sheath provides lubrication as it creates an oil-like substance called synovial fluid which allows for the smooth slip and slide property of the tendon inside the sheath.

To illustrate this, turn your palm upwards and look at your wrist. Move your fingers as if you were typing on a computer or playing a piano. Look at all that movement that occurs at your wrist!

Keep doing that and look at your forearm between the wrist and elbow. Do you see all the movement that is going on? As the muscles located in the upper part of our forearm contract and relax (jump around as we move our fingers), the tendons slide back and forth inside their sheaths and pull our fingers into our palm. In CTS, the smooth back and forth action of our tendons inside their sheaths is disrupted by too much pressure and swelling inside the tunnel (see B, D, & E below). The nerve passes through the carpal tunnel between the floor (transverse carpal ligament) and the bundle of tendons and sheaths and as a result of the swelling, gets squeezed between the ligament and the tendon/sheaths. When any nerve is pinched, numbness or tingling occurs and/or muscle weakness is noticed. When pinched, the median nerve (#9 in C, D, & E below) creates numbness in the 2nd-4th fingers and eventually, weakness in grip and pinch strength.

A. Normal   B. Collapse of the bridge   C. Normal   D. Tenosynovitis   E. Mass (arrow)

The brace or cock-up splint allows the wrist to stay in a neutral / straight position so the pressure on the nerve is minimized. This allows the CTS patient to sleep through the night without waking up with numb, tingling fingers that require shaking or flicking to "wake them up." The brace is usually only worn at night since it's too clumsy to wear during the day and frequently creates more problems when worn while working. Of course, there are many other treatment approaches used by chiropractors which have been previously discussed in prior articles (please refer to prior issues for a list of the many chiropractic treatment approaches).

CTS - Treatment Recommendations

Carpal tunnel syndrome (CTS) is one of the most common causes of pain, loss of work, and work-related disability in the United States. It affects approximately 50 per 1,000 persons in the general population and the average lifetime cost of CTS (including medical bills and lost work time) is estimated to be about $30,000 per each injured worker. In 2003, there were more than 3.8 million visits made to healthcare providers for CTS.

The diagnosis of CTS is based on the patient's complaints, examination findings, and special testing such as electro-diagnostic tests (like Electromyography or EMG). The success or failure of treating CTS rests on the accuracy of the diagnosis. Often, patients with CTS will present after surgery complaining of the same symptoms they had prior to surgery, such as numbness and pain in the index, 3rd and 4th fingers, weak grip, sleep interruptions, and so on, only to find that the median nerve is pinched higher up than the wrist, such as in the neck or elbow.

Treatment failure, as well as an increased likelihood of developing CTS, may also result from the presence of other "risk factors." These include (but are not limited to) advancing age (>50 years old), females > males, and the presence of diabetes and/or obesity, which often coincide. Other risk factors include pregnancy (due to hormonal shifts and fluid retention), certain occupations (highly repetitive), strong family history of CTS, specific medical conditions (like hypothyroidism, autoimmune and rheumatologic diseases), certain types of arthritis, kidney disease, trauma, anatomic predisposition of the wrist and hand (shape and size), infectious diseases, and substance abuse. The difficult thing in treating CTS is when multiple factors exist – like a female over 50 with a highly repetitive job and who is also obese. Obviously, the "best" treatment here would include weight management, and possibly workstation modifications, in addition to the in-office treatment approaches. Patient compliance or following the doctor's recommendations is VERY important such as wearing the wrist splint at night, doing the carpal tunnel stretch exercises, weight management / dietary recommendations, and so on. Therefore, successful treatment for CTS relies on a balance between the patient and provider communicating about ALL the treatment options (surgical and non-surgical) so the patient can make an informed decision. Since each patient is unique, the treatment approach must be tailored to that individual and may require, as previously stated, a number of treatment strategies aimed at patient-specific issues.

Chiropractic is in a unique position for managing the CTS patient. This is because doctors of chiropractic look at the whole person, not just the wrist, and offer the LEAST INVASIVE approach. Many times, there are issues in the neck, shoulder, elbow, and forearm in addition to the wrist/hand that MUST BE carefully assessed in order to obtain a successful, satisfying result for the patient. They also consider the many "risk factors" described above and can assess or coordinate services with other healthcare providers so the many conditions described previously can be properly evaluated. So, the question remains, what do chiropractors do when treating a patient with CTS? Treatment often includes "the usual" such as wrist splinting during sleep, work modifications, and anti-inflammatory approaches (ice cupping, herbal, etc.). Unique to chiropractic are manipulation or adjustments (often to the neck, shoulder, elbow, forearm, wrist, and hand), muscle tendon release techniques (possibly using tools to breakup adhesions, scar tissue, and the like), exercise training for the involved areas including the hand/wrist, as well as dietary strategies for weight management, metabolic syndrome (pre-diabetes), and so on.

Carpal Tunnel Nerve Gliding Exercises

There are many different exercises that can be done for carpal tunnel syndrome (CTS) and we've discussed some of these in the past.

To understand "why" gliding exercises are helpful, let's review the anatomy of the carpal tunnel. There are 9 tendons that move through the narrow carpal tunnel at the wrist. This confined space is literally jammed full and when we move our hands and fingers in a fast, repetitive manner, we produce friction and therefore heat between the tendons that attach the muscles in the forearm to the fingers in the hand. These tendons are in "sheaths" that wrap around the tendon and provide lubrication for the sliding tendon. If the friction/heat builds up too quickly, swelling occurs, which increases the pressure inside the confined space of the carpal tunnel. The median nerve sits on top of all these sheathed tendons and when they expand or swell, the nerve gets pushed up into the roof of the tunnel (the transverse carpal ligament). An analogy would be a river or lake rising to a point where a bridge that goes over the river is eventually engulfed by the rising water. Any object under the bridge would get pushed into the bottom of the bridge (which would represent the median nerve being pinched up against the bridge, or transverse carpal ligament. When nerves are pinched, depending on how much pressure is applied to the nerve, there can be numbness, weakness, pain, and tingling. If the nerve is damaged, the symptoms are more severe. Therefore, in treating CTS, the combination of ice massage over the carpal tunnel (for about 5 minutes or until numb), chiropractic joint manipulation, a splint at night to prevent wrist bending (which increases CT pressure), and EXERCISE are very important. Follow your doctor's recommendation as the when to start the exercises as starting too soon may actually result in a worsening of symptoms!

The concepts behind gliding exercises include: 1. Break up adhesions that form between the sliding tendons and their sheaths; 2. Move blood and other fluids OUT of the tunnel; 3. Improve the range of movement of the wrist and fingers joints. So here they are:

1. **FINGER EXTENSIONS:** a. Hold the arm out straight at shoulder height (near a wall); b. Rotate your arm so the palm faces downwards; c. Bend the wrist backwards as hard as possible by pressing the palm of the hand against the wall; d. Reach over with the opposite hand, grab the thumb and pull back so that a firm "good hurt" stretch is felt in the forearm and HOLD for 5-10 seconds. Repeat this 3 times, pulling the thumb a little harder each time. Repeat this on both sides (so you can see what the difference is in terms of flexibility) 3x/day or as directed.

2. **BEAR CLAW to FULL FIST:** a. Same start position as "1"; b. bend the wrists back & fingers pointing up, so that the palms face away from you and open up the fingers & thumb (the "high 5" position); c. Flex/bend only the tips of your fingers keeping the base of the finger knuckles straight ("Bear Claw"); hold 5 seconds and then repeat a & b but change "c" so that you make a full fist by bending all the hand joints; hold 5 seconds and repeat the entire cycle 3 times (hand open – bear claw – hand open – full fist x3) and repeat multiple times a day or as directed.

Exercises For Carpal Tunnel Syndrome

Carpal tunnel syndrome (CTS) is a common condition resulting in hand and sometimes neck and arm complaints. This can include numbness or tingling in the fingers, leading to dexterity problems such as difficulty buttoning clothing or picking up small objects. An individual with CTS can also experience strength loss / weakness when turning door knobs, opening jars, and even turning the key to start a car. One big problem with CTS is people often wait too long before having it treated thinking it will "…go away" on its own. CTS rarely gets better without some form of treatment and seeing a chiropractor makes perfect sense prior to considering surgical intervention.

So, the question remains, "what can I do for CTS?" There are several things a CTS sufferer can do to help manage their condition. Some risk factors such as gender and age cannot be changed but other factors that may increase pressure inside the carpal tunnel can be alleviated by maintaining a healthy weight, taking mini-breaks at work, modifying the workstation or work activities, wearing a wrist splint at night, and performing exercises to stretch the wrist area.

A study conducted by scientists at the University of Oklahoma found two out of three patients with mild-to-moderate CTS avoided surgery by performing wrist-specific exercises.

Here is one such routine you can try:

- Step A: Extend and stretch both wrists and fingers acutely as if they are in a standing push-up position. Hold for a count of 5.

- Step B: Straighten both wrists and relax fingers.

- Step C: Make a tight fist with both hands.

- Step D: Then, bend both wrists down while keeping the fist. Hold for a count of 5.

- Step E: Straighten both wrists and relax fingers, for a count of 5.

- Step F: Then, let your arms hang loosely at the side and shake them for a few seconds.

This exercise should be repeated 10 times and can be repeated several times a day.

Carpal Tunnel Syndrome (CTS) – A "Typical" Case Example

"I've been working on the line for 13 years and started noticing periodic tingling in my fingers. It didn't last long and I didn't think about it much. It gradually became more frequent and wouldn't go away when I changed my activity or shook my hand or fingers. It started to really grab my attention when I started to drop things out of my hand and couldn't open jars as easily. That's when I decided to see what was wrong. I didn't know who to go to so I went to my family doctor and he diagnosed carpal tunnel syndrome. He gave me a splint to wear at night and some anti-inflammatory drugs that irritated my stomach, so I quit the drugs. The splint helped me sleep and I didn't wake up as often. The doctor was talking about surgery to un-pinch the nerve at my wrist if it didn't get better soon, but I overheard some co-workers talk about seeing a chiropractor for their carpal tunnel problems and how much better they felt so I decided to try it.

"The chiropractor was very thorough and examined my neck, shoulder, elbow as well as my wrist and hand. He indicated that several areas were putting pressure on the nerve that goes into the hand and the pinch was not just at the wrist but higher up in my neck, shoulder and forearm. He said if I wasn't at least 50% better in 4 weeks, we would talk about other tests and treatment options and investigate it further. He worked on my neck, shoulder, elbow, forearm and hand, using manipulations and other methods to loosen it up. He said the nerve was getting pinched by the muscles working too fast and not getting enough rest. He gave me exercises to do several times a day at work to stretch the forearm muscles and had me continue the use of the brace at night. He also taught me how to ice massage the wrist for 5 minutes until it got numb, several times a day and he recommended I use vitamin B6, 50mg, three times a day. After the 3rd week, I started to notice a decrease in the intensity, frequency and duration of numbness and weakness. He had me fill out a Carpal Tunnel Questionnaire and my score improved a lot after the first 4 weeks. He said he may have to evaluate my

workstation and make some modifications, if possible. He asked me a lot about the position of my wrist and hand when I work and didn't seem to like the type of screw driver I was using. He called my boss and asked if a different type of screw driver with a power source and a pistol shaped handle could be tried and it was arranged. That seemed to really make a difference."

Carpal Tunnel Syndrome or CTS, is a common problem that is usually cumulative, slow and gradual in its onset, and can progress to a point where functions like buttoning shirts, threading a needle, and holding a newspaper are greatly affected. People usually don't run to the doctor at the first signs of CTS as the initial symptoms are vague and initially not too impairing. Over time, CTS can become quite severe and often prompts a surgical recommendation, without trying a non-surgical approach first.

There are a number of studies published regarding the chiropractic management of CTS that show these non-surgical methods can be quite successful. One compared medical care consisting of non-steroidal anti-inflammatory drugs and nocturnal wrist splinting to chiropractic care consisting of spine and extremity manipulation, nocturnal wrist splinting, and ultrasound over the wrist. Both treatment approaches were helpful, suggesting the importance of trying either or even both of these non-surgical treatments prior to proceeding to surgery.

Carpal Tunnel Syndrome (CTS) – Exercise Options

There are many exercise options for Carpal tunnel syndrome (CTS). This is because CTS is a "cumulative trauma" condition where repetitive motion results in overuse and subsequent injury to multiple areas in the upper extremities. Most exercises address the forearm, wrist and hand as well as the neck, shoulder, and elbow, depending on the extent of the cumulative injury. Since each case of CTS is unique and individually different from other cases, it is smart to start with basic exercises and add more exercises over time rather than to begin too many exercises at once.

Because CTS is caused most frequently from overusing the hands over time such as a repetitive job or hobby, stretching the inflamed tendons (the string-like attachments of muscles to the bone) in an important objective. There are 4 basic movements of the wrist and the muscles that move the wrist and fingers are located in the forearm and hand. Hence, stretching will take place in these four different directions as overuse injuries or tendonitis is usually not limited only to the carpal tunnel tendons (located on the palm side of the wrist), but usually includes many of the other muscle/tendons on the thumb and/or back side of the wrist. The following are 3 exercises that stretch the wrist/hand on the thumb side, back side, and palm side.

Exercise 1 (for the thumb side of the wrist): START POSITION: Sit or stand with both arms held out straight (elbows, wrists & fingers), thumbs pointing upwards & palms facing each other. MOVEMENT 1: Tuck the thumb into the each palm and grab it with the other 4 fingers making a fist with the thumb inside the fist. MOVEMENT 2: Bend the wrist downwards towards the ground and feel the stretch on the top/thumb side in the wrist and thumb. Hold for 8-10 seconds and repeat many times a day (example once an hour).

Exercise 2 (for the back side of the wrist): START POSITION: Same as above. MOVEMENT 1: Bend (flex) the fingers at the big knuckles (base of the fingers) followed by flexing the wrist. MOVEMENT 2: Using your other hand, pull the back of the hand and apply a gradually increasing stretch until a "good hurt" is achieved on the back side of the forearm, wrist and hand. Hold for 8-10 seconds and repeat many times a day (example once an hour).

Exercise 3

(for the palm side of the wrist): START POSITION: Same as above. MOVEMENT 1: With the fingers pointing downwards, place the palm of the hand on the wall or hook the fingers on the edge of a desk or table's edge and apply a gradual increasing stretch by bending the hooked fingers backwards until the "good hurt" is felt in the forearm palm-side muscles. MOVEMENT 2: Reach over the top with your other hand and grasp your thumb and pull back adding an additional stretch to the tendons that travel through the carpal tunnel. Hold for 8-10 seconds and repeat many times a day (example once an hour).

Done together, these 3 exercises, performed multiple times a day, (especially during work or at times of fast, repetitive arm/hand movements) can act as a "mini-break" from the fast, repetitive work. Chiropractic approaches include training of these and other exercises as well as manipulation/mobilization of the joints including the neck, shoulder, elbow, forearm, wrist and hand, depending on what is needed for each case. Wrist splinting, especially at night, nutritional advice, workstation assessments, also play important roles in the non-surgical care of CTS. We appreciate the opportunity to help you, your family, friends or co-workers who are suffering from CTS. Remember – try this approach first, BEFORE surgery, as this approach carries less risk and, it is frequently all that is needed!

Prompt Treatment Is Best!

Many people suffer from CTS (Carpal Tunnel Syndrome) and unfortunately, often ignore the initial symptoms of numbness or tingling in the hand(s). These early symptoms are typically not too alarming and hence, they often do not raise the level of concern until more intense symptoms occur; such as waking up from sleep due to numbness, dropping items, difficulty buttoning clothing, needing to switch hands when driving, difficulty writing, typing, knitting, as well as work related pain. There may also be fear of job loss associated with CTS, especially in these hard economic times with frequent lay offs, prompting CTS sufferers to postpone initial care. Unfortunately, delaying treatment is associated with a longer recovery time when compared to prompt management which usually results in a quicker, less complicated and more satisfying recovery.

There are many causes and contributing factors of CTS. The most prevalent cause is mechanical irritation from simply moving the hands too fast for too long, without enough rest. Another risk factor is age (over 50 years old). In this era of an aging workforce, this may be a significant issue. Fast, repetitive movements of the arms and hands are often a direct cause and can be appreciated by watching someone knit rapidly and/or performing line work using fast, repetitive movements. If the hands/wrists have to bend in awkward positions to accomplish a work task, or if a tool that is frequently used places pressure in the palm of the hand, these can also contribute to the onset or perpetuation of CTS. Other conditions can also contribute to CTS including inflammatory arthritis like rheumatoid, diabetes, pregnancy, the use of birth control pills, obesity and hypothyroidism.

The management of CTS is case specific, and is dependant on which of the above mentioned causes or contributors are present. Management of any metabolic disorder such as diabetes or hypothyroid is important, especially compliance with taking appropriate medication, when indicated. The management of weight, hormone replacement therapy, and fluid retention all play a roll in CTS management. Ergonomic or job-related management strategies are very important and can include work station modifications so that unnecessary awkward arm/wrist/hand positions can be avoided. This may require moving the item being worked on to a less stressful position, using a different type of tool handle (screw driver, etc.), changing the height or reach distance at which the material is worked on, and taking "mini-breaks" every ½ to 1 hour when the lack of rest is a contributor. Frequently, the combination of pinching a phone between the head and shoulder, typing data into a computer where the monitor is positioned too high or off to one side, and excessive arm motions using a computer mouse can contribute to pinching the nerve in the neck and/or arm, resulting in CTS. Remedies for this situation include the use of a head set, repositioning the computer monitor so that it is in front of the worker, and using a trackball type of mouse to eliminate arm motion can be extremely helpful. Treatment strategies offered by chiropractors include the use of night splinting to avoid awkward wrist/hand positions during sleep. In addition, manual therapy to the wrist and the tight muscles in the front of the forearm, as well as other nerve constriction areas such as the elbow, shoulder, and neck, manipulation of the joints in hand, wrist, elbow, shoulder, and/or neck, depending on what is unique and needed for that patient, and the use of physiological therapeutics such as low level laser light therapy, electrical stimulation, and/or ultrasound have all been shown to offer beneficial effects. Nutritional recommendations include Vitamin B6 (150mg/day), magnesium, calcium, Co-Q10, omega 3 fatty acids and vitamin D3. Reducing glutens (wheat, oats, barley, and rye) is also very important due to the inflammatory response of these foods. Surgery is typically, the last treatment resort and is appropriate, "when all else fails." We welcome you to our clinic and are proud to offer you a non-drug, non-surgical solution for CTS and its disabling symptoms.

FIBROMYALGIA

Fibromyalgia Sleep "Tips"

Last month, we discussed the connection between sleep disturbance and the presence of widespread pain found with fibromyalgia (FM). This month's topic will center on how we can improve our sleep quality with the goal of feeling restored upon waking in the morning!

1) NOISE & LIGHT: Block out noise with earplugs or a sound machine and light with window blinds, heavy curtains, and/or an eye mask. The light emanating from the LED or LCD from TVs, DVRs, or stereos has been found to suppress the pineal gland's melatonin production (the "sleep hormone") and thus can interfere with sleep, so try to keep them away from the bedroom. However, a small night light can assist for nighttime bathroom callings!

2) FOOD: Avoid large meals at least two hours before bedtime. Try a glass of milk, yogurt, or a small protein snack if hunger overcomes you. Milk is unique as it contains the amino acid L-tryptophan, which studies show, helps people sleep!

3) EXERCISE: Aerobic exercise during the day is HIGHLY therapeutic. It reduces stress, reduces pain, reduces depression, and wakes us up! Avoid heavy exercise within three hours before bedtime. Exercise on a REGULAR basis to promote high-quality deep sleep.

4) SLEEP HABITS: Develop good sleeping habits by going to bed at a regular time. Avoid napping in the late afternoon. A "POWER NAP" of no more than 10-15 minutes, ideally about eight hours after waking, is a GOOD THING as it can help you feel refreshed.

5) MENTAL TASKS: Avoid mentally stimulating activity one hour before bedtime to calm the brain.

6) MENTAL CLARITY: Avoid bedtime worries. Try NOT to think about things that are upsetting. Substitute positive thoughts, experiences, and/or visualize favorite hobbies that free up the mind. Try to avoid discussing emotional issues before bedtime.

7) PETS: They are GREAT companions but NOT in the bed at night! Not only can pets kicking and moving disturb rest, their dander can stir up allergies and interfere with sleep.

8) TEMPERATURE: A well-ventilated and temperature controlled (54-74° F or 12.2-23.3° Celsius) bedroom is "key."

9) BEDROOM "RULES": The bedroom is for two things: physical intamacy and sleeping. If you wake up in the middle of the night, go to another room and read a book or watch TV until you feel sleepy.

10) AVOID STIMULANTS: AVOID nicotine, caffeine, coffee, chocolate, tea, soft drinks, and various over-the-counter or prescription medications in the late evening, unless under instruction from your physician.

11) RELAXATION TECHNIQUES: Try one (there are many) and practice it at bedtime.

12) REFRAIN FROM DRINKING ALCOHOL: Alcohol is a nervous system depressant and can HELP you fall asleep, BUT a rebound withdrawal can cause nightmares and night sweats. Avoid this close to bedtime (switch to water!).

Fibromyalgia and Sleep — Is There a Connection?

Is there a connection between fibromyalgia (FM) and sleep disturbance? Let's take a look!

FM is a condition that causes widespread pain and stiffness in muscles and joints. Patients with FM often experience chronic daytime fatigue and some type of sleep problems like getting to sleep, staying asleep, and/or feeling restored in the morning upon waking. The National Institutes of Health estimates between 80-90% of those diagnosed with FM are middle-aged women, although it can affect men and happen at any age. As little as 10-20 years ago, it was hard to find a doctor who "believed" in FM, and it was common for the patient to be told that their pain "was all in their head." FM has now been studied to the point that we know it is a real condition, and it affects between 2-6% of the general population around the world.

It is well established that sleep disturbance frequently occurs after surgery, which usually normalizes as time passes. One study used a group of healthy women who were deprived of sleep (particularly slow wave sleep) for three days to see if there was a link between sleep disturbance and pain. Results confirmed that the women experienced a decrease in pain tolerance and increased levels of discomfort and fatigue after three days—the same symptoms found among FM sufferers!

Fibromyalgia may have NO known cause, or it can be triggered by other conditions such as repetitive stress injuries, car crash injuries, and other forms of trauma. FM also appears to run in families though it's still NOT clear if this is a true genetic link or caused by shared environmental factors. Some feel FM is a rheumatoid condition, and though FM is NOT a true form of arthritis, it has been found that people with arthritis are more likely to have FM.

FM sufferers frequently suffer from conditions such as irritable bowel syndrome, chronic fatigue syndrome, migraine headaches, arthritis, lupus, and major depressive disorders.

Approximately 20% of FM patients have depression and/or anxiety disorders, and a link between chronic pain and depression exists and seems to play a role in people's perception of pain.

Because conditions such as sleep apnea can result in symptoms similar to FM, it's recommended that patients suspected of FM keep a sleep/sleepiness diary in order to rule out sleep apnea as a cause for their condition.

There are many "tips" for improving sleep quality, which we will dive into next month, as these may prove VERY HELPFUL in the management of FM!

Fibromyalgia "Diet" – Is There Such a Thing?

Folks suffering with fibromyalgia (FM) commonly complain that certain foods can make their symptoms worse. How common is this? One study reported 42% of FM patients found that certain foods worsened their symptoms!

Because FM affects each person differently, there is no ONE FM diet or, "…one size fits all" when it comes to eating "right" for FM. Patients with FM usually find out by trial and error which foods work vs. those that consistently don't. However, remembering which foods do what can be a challenge so FIRST, make a three column FOOD LOG with the following headings: BETTER, NO CHANGE, WORSE. This will allow you to QUICKLY review the list as a memory refresher.

According to Dr. Ginevra Liptan, medical director of the Frida Center for Fibromyalgia (Portland, OR) and author of Figuring Out Fibromyalgia: Current Science and the Most Effective Treatments, there are some common trends she's observed through treating FM patients. Here are some of her recommendations:

PAY ATTENTION TO HOW FOOD MAKES YOU FEEL: It is quite common to have "sensitivities" to certain foods, but this is highly variable from person to person. Examples of problematic foods/ingredients include: MSG (commonly used in Chinese food), other preservatives, eggs, gluten, and dairy. Dr. Liptan HIGHLY recommends the food journal approach! She also recommends including a note about the type of symptoms noticed with each "WORSE" food, as symptoms can vary significantly.

ELIMINATE CERTAIN FOODS: If you suspect a certain food may be problematic, try an elimination challenge diet. That means STOP eating that food for six to eight weeks and then ADD it back into your diet and see how you feel. Remember, FM sufferers frequently have irritable bowel syndrome, also known as IBS, and this approach can be REALLY HELPFUL! Food allergies may be part of the problem, and your doctor may refer you for a consult with an allergist and/or a dietician. They will also discuss the "anti-inflammatory diet" with you.

EAT HEALTHY: In general, your diet should emphasize fruits and vegetables and lean protein. Pre-prepare food so you have something "healthy" to reach for rather than a less healthy snack when you're hungry and tired. Consider "pre-washed" and pre-cut up vegetables; try quinoa rather than pasta. Consume anti-fatigue foods and eat multiple small meals daily vs. one to two large meals. Protein snacks (like a hardboiled egg or oatmeal – GLUTEN FREE) help a lot! Eat breakfast and include protein. Also, GET ENOUGH SLEEP (at least seven to eight hours and be consistent)!

SUPPLEMENTS: Consider a good general multi-vitamin, calcium and magnesium, omega-3 fatty acids, vitamin D3, and Co-Enzyme Q10. There are others, but this represents a great place to start. Remember to check any medication you may be taking with these/any suggestions before taking supplements!

Dietary Strategies to Treat Fibromyalgia

Fibromyalgia (FM) is a common condition that affects about five million Americans, often between ages 20 and 45 years old. FM is very difficult to diagnose primarily because there is no definitive test like there is for heart, liver, or kidney disease. Equally challenging is the ability to effectively treat FM as there are frequently other conditions that co-exist with FM that require special treatment considerations. Typically, each FM case is unique with a different group of symptoms and therefore, each person requires individualized care.

Fibromyalgia symptoms can include generalized pain throughout the body that can vary from mild to severely disabling, extreme fatigue, nausea/flu-like symptoms, brain "fog" ("fibro-fog"), depression and/or anxiety, sleeping problems and feeling un-refreshed in the mornings, headaches, irritable bowel syndrome, morning stiffness, painful menstrual cramps, numbness or tingling (arms/hands, legs/feet), tender points, urinary pain or burning, and more!

So, let's talk about ways to improve your FM-related symptoms through dietary approaches. When the FM symptom group includes gut trouble (bad/painful gas, bloating, and/or constipation), it's not uncommon to have an imbalance between the "good" vs. the "bad" bacteria, yeast, and problems with digestion or absorption. Think of management as a "Four Step" process for the digestive system:

1. REMOVE HARMFUL TOXINS: Consider food allergy testing to determine any foods the FM patient has a sensitivity for. Frequently, removing gluten, dairy, eggs, bananas, potatoes, corn, and red meat can benefit the FM patient. The use of anti-fungal and / or anti-bacterial botanicals (as opposed to drug approaches such as antibiotics) can be highly effective. A low allergy-potential diet consisting of fish, poultry, certain vegetables, legumes, fruits, rice, and olive and coconut oil is usually a good choice.

2. IMPROVE DIGESTIVE FUNCTION: The presence of bloating and gas is usually indicative of poor digestion, and the use of a digestive enzyme with every meal can be highly effective!

3. RESTORE THE "GOOD" BACTERIA: Probiotics (with at least 20-30 billion live organisms) at each meal are often necessary to improve the "good" gut bacteria population, which will likely also improve immune function.

4. REPAIR THE GUT: If the gut wall is damaged, nutrients like l-glutamine, fish oils, and n-acetyl-d-glucosamine may help repair it.

This process will take several months, and some of these approaches may have to be continued over the long term. Doctors of chiropractic are trained in nutritional counseling and can help you in this process. As an added benefit, many FM sufferers find the inclusion of chiropractic adjustments to be both symptomatically relieving and energy producing.

Can I PREVENT Fibromyalgia?

Fibromyalgia (FM) is a common cause for chronic pain (pain that lasts three or more months) and afflicts 4% of the general population in the United States! FM commonly affects the muscles and soft tissues – not the joints (like arthritis); however, many FM sufferers are mistakenly diagnosed with arthritis, so it may take years before they get an accurate diagnosis. There are NO known accurate diagnostic tests for FM, which is another reason for a delayed diagnosis.

In order to answer the question, "Can fibromyalgia be prevented?" we must first find the cause of FM. There are two types of FM: PRIMARY and SECONDARY. Primary FM occurs for no known reason, while secondary FM can be triggered by a physical event such as a trauma (e.g., car accident), an emotional event or a stressful situation (e.g., loss of a child), and/or a medical event such as a condition like irritable bowel syndrome, rheumatoid arthritis, or systemic lupus erythymatosus (SLE). Any condition that carries chronic or long-lasting symptoms can trigger FM, and some argue that the lack of being able to get into the deep sleep stage may be at the core of triggering FM since sleep disorders are a common finding in FM sufferers!

The "KEY" to managing FM has consistently been and probably always will be EXERCISE and SLEEP. So, if FM is preventable, daily exercise and getting the "right kind" of sleep are very important ways that may reduce the likelihood for developing the condition! Since emotions play a KEY ROLE in the cause and/or effect of FM, applying skills that keep life's stressors in check is also important. This list can include hobbies like reading a good book, playing and/or listening to music, or meditation. The combination of exercise with mindful meditation using approaches like Tai Chi, Yoga, Qi Gong, and others has had positive impacts on FM patients such as improved balance and stability, reduced pain, enhanced mental clarity, and generally improved quality of life. Managing physical conditions that are associated with FM (such as irritable bowel syndrome, rheumatoid arthritis, or systemic lupus erythymatosus) is also important in managing and/or preventing FM.

Another management strategy of FM is diet. As most patients with FM will agree, certain foods help and others make the FM symptoms worse. In a survey published in the Journal of Cinlical Rheumatology, 42% of FM patients reported certain foods exacerbated their symptoms. Of course, each individual case is unique, so keeping a food log or journal can be very helpful to determine dietary "friends" vs. "enemies." The first step is to eliminate certain foods for four to six weeks, such as dairy and/or gluten. Most patients report a significant improvement in energy (less fatigue) while some report less pain when problem foods are elimated from their diet. Generally, a diet rich in fruits, vegetables, and lean proteins can have a positive impact on the FM patient. Consider eating multiple small meals vs. two or three large meals during the day, as this can keep blood sugar levels more stable and reduce fatigue.

So back to the question, can fibromyalgia be prevented? Maybe...maybe not. Since the medical community doesn't know the exact cause, it's hard to answer this question. However, being proactive and implementing the strategies used to better manage FM may help in preventing it as well!

How Are Fibromyalgia Exercises Different?

For some people, fibromyalgia (FM) can make life miserable. In some cases, it can be so bad a person will spend the majority of the day in bed! When FM is this intense, exercises MUST be tailored accordingly – like starting out with exercises that can be done in bed! Initially, you may only be able to exercise for one to two minutes, but slowly, your tolerance will improve! Here are some "steps" that one may consider for implementing exercise into the FM sufferer's lifestyle.

STEP 1: POSITIVE ATTITUDE: It's easier said than done to have a "positive attitude" about anything, much less exercise when FM has its grip on you! In fact, depression is a BIG problem with most FM patients. Both studies and experience have shown that exercise is one of the most effective ways to treat FM. This is because exercise benefits ALL of our bodily functions from the brain to the heart, lungs, muscle/joints, and gut! It even benefits symptoms like fatigue, depression, and sleep problems. It helps bone density, improves balance, increases strength, controls weight, and reduces stress! As one FM patient said, "...this may be the last thing you feel like doing, but you have to believe that it really does help."

STEP 2: START SLOWLY: Just like training for a marathon, you DON'T begin with a ten-mile run! You have to increase the distance and pace gradually. With FM, a person needs to steadily work into exercise because the post-exercise pain (that you should expect initially) may scare them away from continuing and/or make them even more hesitant about trying it again. Consider an initial one-to-two minute routine and gradually add more time and distance to that, ramping up the intensity and duration of exercise over time! Remember, it may take 15 weeks to reach a 30-minute goal of treadmill walking, elliptical use, or swimming. Consider taking stairs, doing household chores, grocery shopping, and gardening/yard work as part of your fitness routine. It doesn't have to be a formal exercise program!

STEP 3: LISTEN TO YOUR BODY: Even if you were very active before FM entered your life, you must learn not push it beyond the "reasonable boundaries" of your usual activity tolerance. Take breaks when necessary and closely monitor how you feel. Your goal is to AVOID FRUSTRATION by NOT over-exercising! Keep track of what you do and how you feel so that you can refer back to such information when needed.

STEP 4: EXERCISE DAILY: Make it a point to walk. Walk the dog (or your neighbor's), take the stairs, park further away from stores, and INCLUDE these activities as part of your workout! When you say, "I worked out today," you don't have to explain yourself to everyone! Consider cycling, walking/running, low-impact yoga or Palates classes, or light weight-lifting. A local gym or class may be a perfect match for what you are looking for!

STEP 5: MODIFY THE WORKOUT: Mix it up so it's not boring! Figure out when you feel best and exercise then. For many FM patients, this is between 10am and 3pm. Include some stretches, balance tasks, vary the stride and/or speed, ease into strength training, pace yourself, and rest when needed.

STEP 6: BE PATIENT: This cannot be overemphasized as it's easy to get frustrated. It can take up to six months before the FM patient may start to feel a change in their symptoms! Patiently work towards realistic goals – Exercise is the #1 best long-term FM treatment method!

The "TOP 10" FACTS of Fibromyalgia!

What are the ten most important attributes of fibromyalgia (FM)? Let's take a look!

1. FM definition : It's characterized by widespread muscular pain and tenderness (in all four of the body's quadrants) that's NOT caused by inflammation or joint damage.

2. FM can be primary or secondary : Secondary FM is caused by something else (often after trauma) in association with another disorder like rheumatoid arthritis (RA), irritable bowel syndrome (IBS), lupus, chronic fatigue syndrome, and more. Primary FM has no known association with another condition.

3. FM is OFTEN chronic : Because FM is diagnosed by EXCLUDING other conditions, it's often left undiagnosed for years! To further complicate this, when a person has a diagnosed condition such as Lyme disease, RA, etc., those conditions get all the attention and FM is left undiagnosed. In fact, the National Fibromyalgia Association reports that it takes about an average of five years to get an accurate diagnosis of FM!

4. Sleep & Chronic Fatigue : A reported 90% of FM patients suffer from severe fatigue or a sleep disorder. Non-restorative sleep contributes significantly to fatigue and poor cognitive function, and is a hallmark of FM making it an important problem to address in treatment.

5. FM Symptoms are many : Headache, IBS, memory problems, TMD (jaw pain), pelvic pain, noise-light-temperature sensitivities, restless leg syndrome (RLS), depression, and anxiety are ALL associated issues with FM (more reasons for a delayed diagnosis and treatment challenges)!

6. FM includes both physical and psychological aspects : One study of 307 FM patients followed over an eleven-year time frame found that 33% had severe physical and psychological

problems, another 1/3 had mild issues with both, and the last third had only mild physical symptoms.

7. F M is HIGHLY VARIABLE : With the widespread pain, variable disability rates, variable physical and psychological aspects (see #6 above), and symptom/condition variability (see #5 above), a treatment approach to manage FM must be individualized! There is no "recipe" for managing FM!

8. FM Tests : There are none! Diagnosing FM relies on the patient's history of widespread pain and associated disabilities more than the physical exam, blood tests, and x-rays which are used to help "rule-out" other disorders.

9. FM Treatment : The "best" management strategies for FM include a multi-disciplinary "team" of providers including primary care (medications), chiropractic (manual therapy, nutrition, exercise training), clinical psychology (depression/anxiety management), and other forms of treatment such as massage therapy, acupuncture, and meditation / relaxation therapy. Programs that are individualized work the best! The patient MUST BE an active participant who is willing to do the work!

10. "Stats" about FM : First of all, it's common! It affects women more than men, and about 2-4% of the population overall. What is left out of the stats is the intensity of symptoms, how well each patient responds to the different management strategies, and the patient's coping skills with this chronic, sometimes totally disabling condition (see #6 above). Other "facts" about FM include: increased "substance P" (a chemical that increases nerve sensitivity), decreased blood flow to the thalamus (brain), hormone imbalances, low levels of serotonin and tryptophan, and abnormal cytokine function....and more!

REMEMBER as stated in #9, the "team" approach yields the BEST RESULTS!

Fibromyalgia – "How Do I Know If I Have It?"

Fibromyalgia (FM) is a condition where widespread generalized pain limits a person's ability to function, sometimes to the point of complete disability. This month, we'll look at identifying markers that may be used to determine whether a patient has FM or not.

Chronic pain that arises from the muscles and joints affects nearly 20% of the adult population, with the highest percentages found among females and those in lower income brackets. It is very challenging to determine "the cause" of chronic pain, probably because it is influenced by and interacts with various physical, emotional, psychological, and social factors. Several studies have reportedly shown that the levels of certain neurotransmitters (chemicals that help our nerves transmit information) including serotonin, glutamate, lactate, and pyruvate are elevated in patients with localized chronic myalgias (like FM) and therefore may be potential biomarkers for various conditions causing chronic pain. Unfortunately, elevations in these potential markers are not specific or unique to FM.

However, researchers have identified muscle alterations in in fibromyalgia / chronic widespread pain patients. More studies are needed to confirm these findings before they have the potential for use as a diagnostic criteria for FM.

For the time being, in order to establish a diagnosis of FM, we must rely on the following:

1) The presence of widespread pain by using the "Widespread Pain Index" or WPI.

2) Determining the severity of the symptoms by using the "Symptom Severity Score" or SS score of which there are two parts:

• Scoring fatigue, waking un-refreshed, and cognitive symptoms using a 0-3 scale, 3 representing the most severe or disturbing of these daily functions.

• Adding up additional symptoms associated with FM, resulting in a 0-3 range depending on the number of the "other symptoms."

Using the WPI and the SS scores, FM can be identified if one of the following two situations has been present for three or more months:

• WPI score > 7 and SS score > 5

• WPI score between 3 and 6 and SS score > 9

Fibromyalgia and the Importance of Sleep

One of the most frustrating symptoms of fibromyalgia (FM) is the inability to get a good night's sleep! Recently, at a Harvard-sponsored conference on the subject of pain, it was stated that "...no one should have to live in constant pain with what is known about pain management in this day and age (paraphrased)." Many attendees agreed that improving sleep quality may be the #1 way to improve the quality of life for patients with widespread pain. So the question is, what can be done to improve the sleep cycle for all of us, not only the fibromyalgia patient? Let's take a look!

The importance of sleep has long been discussed as being not only key in managing the FM patient, but some experts even suspect it's the probable cause of the disorder itself. It has been found that we must get at least four hours of continuous sleep in order to reach a deep sleep stage, and only at this level of sleep can we fully relax. If we can't get to that deep sleep stage, our muscles (and mind) can't fully relax and over time, the gradually increasing tightness may result in pain and the vicious cycle continues to chip away at the quality of life of the FM patient.

Exciting new research from the United Kingdom reports that for those over age 50, non-restorative sleep – the type where you wake up tired, foggy, and listless - is STRONGLY tied to widespread pain, the "hallmark" of FM. The researchers also report that anxiety, memory loss, and poor physical health are linked to widespread pain in older adults. In the journal Arthritis & Rheumatology, author Dr. John McBeth wrote that musculoskeletal pain becomes more common with aging and affects four out of five seniors on a daily basis! Widespread pain is a KEY FEATURE of FM, which also includes fatigue and tenderness in muscles, joints, tendons, and other soft tissues. It is estimated that about 5 million American adults are affected by FM with women being affected four times more often than men (for reasons unknown). FM can occur insidiously (for no known reason) or secondary to an injury or illness.

After studying a group of 4,300 adults (> age 50) of which 2,700 had some pain but not widespread pain, Dr. McBeth and his colleagues found several factors that can increase an older individual's risk of developing widespread pain. At the start of the study, participants completed questionnaires about pain, mental and physical health, lifestyle and health behaviors, medical conditions, and more. After three years, they were reassessed in a similar manner and 19% reported NEW widespread pain. This included 25% of participants who initially reported some pain and 8% who reported no pain at the study's start. The most important link for the development of widespread pain was non-restorative sleep. Other links included pain status, anxiety, physical health-related quality of life, and some form of cognitive complaint (such as memory loss). They also note that brainwave studies of FM sufferers often show the inability to reach deep sleep. Moreover, in an experiment where healthy volunteers were woken during each period of deep sleep, a number of them soon developed typical signs and symptoms of FM!

Chiropractic care includes treatment methods that reduces pain and muscle spasm and as a result, frequently improves an interrupted sleep pattern. Doctors of chiropractic are also STRONG ADVOCATES of home exercise and typically offer in-office training. Before attempting drugs with significant side effects, you owe it to yourself to include chiropractic care in your FM management "team!"

Fibromyalgia – Drugs vs. Herbs & Supplements?

Fibromyalgia (FM) is characterized by a whole body, widespread pain that affects millions of people and continues to be a challenge for both doctors and patients to manage. This is probably because there is no one cause that can be clearly identified with the onset of FM. The "best" approach to managing FM requires a "team" of healthcare providers and a multi-modal treatment approach including (but not limited to): medications, chiropractic adjustments, exercise training, relaxation techniques, proper nutrition/diet, and structured sleep habits. The focus of this month's article is on various oral treatment options, both prescription and non-prescription varieties that focus on deep muscle pain, sleep problems, anxiety, and depression.

DRUGS : The following is a partial list of medications commonly prescribed for FM, according to WebMD. Please consult with your medical doctor as to which medication(s) may be best for you, if any: Cymbalta, Lyrica, and Savella.

HERBS/SUPPLEMENTS : Last month, we discussed getting enough vitamin D, avoiding food additives such as MSG and aspartame, consuming omega 3 fatty acids, avoiding caffeine, eating veggies, taking anti-oxidants (such as vitamin A, C, and E, and coenzyme Q10), and avoiding gluten. Additional considerations include:

1. 5-HTP: This is a "building block" for a powerful brain neurotransmitter called serotonin, which is thought to play a significant role in reducing FM-related pain, reducing depression, and helping to facilitate sleep – especially deep sleep! One study reported improvement in depression, anxiety, and insomnia as

well as FM-related pain. This is usually well-tolerated by FM patients.

2. Melatonin: This is a natural hormone used to induce drowsiness and improve sleep patterns. It may also be effective in reducing pain associated with FM. This is regarded as being safe with few-to-no side effects, though it may cause daytime sleepiness for some so don't drive or operate heavy machinery until you see how it affects you.

3. St. John's Wart: Though NOT specific or unique in FM treatment, it is often used to treat depression, which is a common FM symptom and therefore, may be helpful. Several studies found this to be more effective than placebo and equally effective as some antidepressants called "tricyclics" in those with mild-to-moderate depression. Other studies found similar results when compared to selective SSRI antidepressants such as Prozac or Zoloft. It is usually well-tolerated with the most common side effects including stomach upset, skin reactions, and fatigue. This reportedly should NOT be mixed with other antidepressants or other supplements.

4. SAM-e: How this exactly works in the body remains unknown, but some feel this natural supplement increases serotonin and dopamine levels (two brain neurotransmitters). Studies support mood improvement and increased restful sleep but it is not significantly beneficial for FM pain reduction or FM-related depression. Additional studies are needed.

5. L-Carnitine: L-Carnitine intake has been linked to FM-related pain relief and general mental health benefits.

6. Probiotics: These "good guy" bacteria or yeast supplements may assist in digestive disorders such as IBS (irritable bowel syndrome), which is commonly associated with FM. Other uses include diarrhea management and urinary tract and female genital tract infections.

7. Other herbs/supplements that may help FM include: Echinacea, black cohosh, cayenne, lavender, milk thistle, and B vitamins. Caution is recommended with using herbs during pregnancy, with children, the elderly, those with immune system deficiency, and those taking a blood thinner.

Food and Fibromyalgia

Fibromyalgia (FM) is a chronic disease that results in generalized pain spread out over the body and affects over 5 million people in the United States alone. Because no one has yet determined the cause of FM, both the diagnosis as well as the treatment poses a big challenge because it's basically a trial and error approach. Dr. Kathleen Holton, the lead author of Potential Dietary Links in Central Sensitization in Fibromyalgia, states that only about 30% of fibromyalgia symptoms improve with the use of the medications that are currently on the market. This is a big reason why FM patients turn to alternative treatments, many of which include dietary approaches. Certain foods can make FM worse, and in fact, up to 42% of FM patients have verified this! Dr. Holton has found the following five recommendations can offer fibromyalgia patients significant benefits:

1. Vitamin D: Vitamin D is hard to get through diet alone, and it's frequently referred to as "the sunshine vitamin" because that's where it is most readily obtained. Some of the symptoms of FM such as bone and muscle pain are mimicked by vitamin D deficiency, and taking vitamin D has been found to reduce these symptoms. This means that ALL patients with FM should have a vitamin D screen through a simple blood test. One study showed that the dosage of pain killers had to be doubled in order to get the same beneficial effects in patients who are vitamin D deficienct. Winter months are an especially challenging time for vitamin D deficiency!

2. Avoid Additives: Common food additives such as MSG (monosodium glutamate) and aspartame can act as "excitotoxins" (chemicals that increase pain sensitivity). Reducing these additives can result in decreased pain in FM patients!

3. Fish is good! Omega 3 fatty acids are strong anti-inflammatory agents that help prevent cardiovascular disease and can be found in walnuts, flaxseed, and fatty fish. A 2007 study reported that symptoms including morning stiffness and painful/tender joints significantly improved after just three months of omega 3 fatty acid supplementation.

4. Avoid caffeine! This is important since FM patients often turn to caffeine to keep them awake during the day, but this can backfire by keeping them up at night! Caffeine (especially when consumed later in the day) can disrupt sleep schedules.

5. Eat your veggies! Scientists have reported that oxidative stress may be a cause of FM symptoms. Oxidative stress occurs when the body fails to produce antioxidants ("the "good guys") to fight off the cell damaging-free radicals (the "bad guys") in the body. Most fruits and veggies are loaded with important anti-oxidants such as vitamins A, C, and E, which fight off free radicals. That's NOT to say that meat is bad, as it's a great source for iron and vitamin B12, which are also important for keeping the pain processing part of our nervous system healthy. Consider an anti-inflammatory diet that emphasizes fruits, vegetables, lean meats (preferably grass-fed beef). It's also recommended that FM patients avoid gluten as it can lead to low-grade inflammation that can worsen their symptoms.

We will help guide you in the process of diet and supplementation in addition to managing you with many other FM effective chiropractic services! Remember, the best FM management outcome is obtained through a TEAM approach!

Commonly Asked Questions about Fibromyalgia

WHAT IS FIBROMYALGIA? FM is a relatively common chronic disorder where widespread pain, diffuse tenderness, and potentially a host of other symptoms may be present. The word "fibromyalgia" is derived from the Latin term "fibro" (fibrous tissue) and the Greek term "myo" for muscle and "algia" for pain. Even though FM is often described as an arthritis-type of condition, it does NOT cause inflammation of the joints, muscles, or other tissues as is observed with some types of arthritis. However, FM does "look" like arthritis in that FM can cause significant pain that can interfere with a person's tolerance to daily activities, including work.

WHO GETS FM? It has been reported that FM affects five million Americans ages 18 and older. For unknown reasons, between 80-90% of those affected are women, but men and children can also develop FM. Most people are diagnosed during their middle years. Several studies have reported that women with a positive family history of FM are more likely to develop FM, but it remains unclear if this is from a shared environment vs. a true heredity issue, or both. Currently, researchers are looking at variations in certain genes that cause some people to be more sensitive to stimuli, which may lead to pain syndromes like FM. People with rheumatic diseases (such as rheumatoid arthritis, lupus, or ankylosing spondylitis – a special type of spinal arthritis) may be more likely to have FM as well.

WHAT CAUSES FM? Even though no one REALLY knows why some people develop FM and others do not, we have learned that FM is linked to the central nervous system. There are two types of FM: Primary (no known cause) and Secondary (occurs with a known underlying condition). Secondary FM has been associated with a physical/emotional stress or traumatic event such as a motor vehicle accident, and some develop FM after sustaining a repetitive motion injury or after an illness. In primary FM, it seems to develop spontaneously with no known cause or associated condition.

HOW IS FM TREATED? Treatment is challenging as not all doctors are familiar with FM and may not even "believe" it's real (they may think it's depression or all in the patient's head). It is therefore BEST to find a "TEAM" of healthcare providers knowledgeable about FM and willing to work with you. This team may include primary care doctors, chiropractors, physical therapists, clinical psychologists, and perhaps rheumatologists, among others. Massage therapists, acupuncturists, and nutritional therapists can also be part of the multi-dimensional treatment approach. However, the MOST important team member is YOU because keeping track of sleep hours, exercise amounts, diet, and knowing when to rest are critical for a good treatment outcome. You can guide us in finding care that works, what doesn't, and at what "dose" feels best for you. Focusing on "control" rather than "cure" is important so you do not get too discouraged during the treatment process.

Tests for Fibromyalgia?

Wouldn't it be nice if you could just tell your chiropractor, primary care doctor, nurse practitioner, or physician assistant about how you're feeling and have the condition easily diagnosed and treated? With fibromyalgia (FM), it NEVER works that way! Some doctors even think FM is a mental issue and don't believe it's a "real" condition. Others over-diagnose everyone with FM and place them on medications that sometimes carry side effects that are worse than the condition. Let's take a look at the diagnostic criteria for FM and discuss what you might expect in regards to tests....

The Diagnostic Guidelines for Fibromyalgia currently state three things: 1) Pain that is widespread in all four quadrants of your body. 2) Pain that has been present for at least three months. 3) There are no other diseases causing these symptoms. In other words, a patient's health history can satisfy the first two criteria and a physical examination and BLOOD TESTS help us rule out other diseases that can cause similar symptom-producing conditions. A commonly ordered blood test is a "CBC" (complete blood count), which tells us if you have an infection (elevated white blood cells – WBCs) or if you are anemic (low red blood cells – RBCs, low hemoglobin, which makes the blood red). Other tests may look for signs of rheumatoid arthritis, gout, a prior strep infection, lupus, inflammation, or Lyme disease. NONE of these tests tell us if you have FM, but they do help us determine if you have some other underlying condition that may be participating in the symptom picture.

However, there is a NEW blood test that may predict fibromyalgia that was introduced in October of 2013 at the annual meeting of the American College of Rheumatology. EpicGenetics of Santa Monica, CA calls it the "FM/a" test, and it's being described as "…objective, very accurate, and definitive." Because of its high cost ($744) and short track record, it's currently being used primarily in the difficult-to-diagnose cases. The test works by measuring proteins in the body that lessen pain (which were found to be low in FM patients). Researchers ran this test on 100 lupus patients, 98 RA patients, 160 FM patients and 119 healthy patients and found it positive in 93% of KNOWN FM patients and negative 89% of non-FM patients! Because this was presented at a conference and not yet "peer reviewed" (published in a medical journal), these findings are "preliminary" and must be interpreted with caution.

A simple/FREE "screen" called the "Widespread Pain Index" ("Google" it) contains two main parts: 1) A pain diagram where you can check off the body parts that hurt; 2a) a Symptom Severity Score where you indicate your level of symptom severity over the past week and 2b) where you check off "Other Symptoms" from a list. There is a scoring method that is simple and described on the form that result in two numbers to determine if you meet the "diagnostic criteria." We recommend starting with this approach. Print off the form, fill it out and score it yourself, bring that into our clinic, and then ask about your specific case. The MOST important part of this process is the third criteria discussed above: ruling out other conditions (we MUST see you!).

Chiropractic is "A MUST" on the management "TEAM" for FM patients, and we're happy to keep you INFORMED of your diagnostic and treatment options!

The Diagnosis and Misdiagnosis of Fibromyalgia

Fibromyalgia (FM) is a condition that the medical community has long had difficulty defining. As stated last month, FM is often considered a "musculoskeletal disorder" (MSK) because of the aches and pains it produces in the muscles and joints. However, this is not really accurate since FM includes many other symptoms beyond just severe muscle pain, such as extreme fatigue, mental fog, sleep disorders, irritable bowel, and more. As such, "misdiagnosis" is more common than an accurate diagnosis when it comes the FM. Let's take a closer look!

FM is described as a "syndrome," meaning it includes multiple complaints and findings that commonly occur together such as (but not limited to) widespread pain, decreased pain tolerance or threshold, multiple tender points, incapacitating fatigue, anxiety, and/or depression. Though the intensity of these symptoms can vary, persistent and chronic fatigue is one of the most common complaints, second only to the whole body deep muscle aches. Unlike "normal" fatigue, the type of fatigue, weakness, and exhaustion associated with FM often leads to social isolation, and as a result, anxiety and/or depression.

The reason WHY FM is so difficult to diagnose is that: 1) These same symptoms are found in many other conditions and, 2) There is no one test that can diagnose FM like a blood test or x-ray. The diagnosis process must RULE OUT all the other conditions that present with similar symptoms. Hence, blood tests are used to rule out anemia or hypothyroid (for fatigue), inflammatory arthritis, and Lyme disease. Sleep studies are used

173

to rule out sleep apnea (which can co-exist with FM). X-rays are used to rule out a bone or joint cause of the patient's muscle pain. Many diseases or conditions have a pattern of complaints, but FM doesn't consistently follow a similar presentation. There are so many different degrees of FM and the symptoms include so many different systems of the body that FM sufferers often have to go from doctor to doctor before they find one willing to take the time needed to properly assess for fibromyalgia. Some doctors firmly believe there is no such thing as FM stating that "...it's all in the head!" This can only adds to the frustration, anxiety, and depression for the FM sufferer.

Common misdiagnoses include (but are not limited to) depression, inflammatory arthritis (like rheumatoid or lupus), chronic myofascial pain syndrome, or chronic fatigue syndrome. Conditions commonly associated with FM may include some of the above as well as irritable bowel syndrome (IBS), thyroid deficiency, and others, which only makes the diagnosis of FM even more challenging!

Some doctors and researchers use the term "primary FM" for FM that is not caused by something else vs. "secondary FM" where something like a trauma (eg., car accident), IBS, or an inflammatory arthritis either precedes the start of FM symptoms or is closely associated with its onset. The important point is that FM is unique and it must be properly diagnosed so accurate and effective treatment can be administered. The diagnostic Guidelines for FM include three main things: 1) Widespread pain in all four body quadrants; 2) At least three months of symptoms; and 3) No other disease is causing these symptoms. You can expect us to check for the following: 1) Widespread pain; 2) Trigger point evaluation; 3) Ask about fatigue; 4) Ask about sleep disturbances; 5) Ask about stress levels; and 6) Ask about depression. Proper treatment is often best approached with a "team" consisting of chiropractic, primary care, clinical psychology and/or counseling, and sometimes others.

Fibromyalgia: The Top 10 Most Common Signs

Fibromyalgia (FM) causes widespread pain to an estimated 5.8 million Americans. FM is considered a "musculoskeletal disorder" even though many of the symptoms include other systems, especially the gastrointestinal system, as conditions such as IBS (irritable bowel syndrome) often co-exist. It is thought that FM is a disorder that amplifies the manner in which the brain processes pain, making the body's pain receptors hypersensitive. For example, FM can result in a 3/10 pain level (normally tolerated) being amplified to 7 or 8/10, enough to interfere with daily activities. FM often follows some type of severe physical or mental trauma, such as a car accident, surgery, or a significant psychological stress. The widespread pain results in fatigue, sleep deprivation, depression, and more. The following are ten of the most common symptoms associated with FM:

1. Pain : This is the primary symptom, and it is typically widespread/whole body but doesn't necessarily occur all at once. It can flair at times of stress, weather changes, sleep schedule change, and it can be achy, stabbing, burning, tingling, pins/needles, or a mix.

2. Sensitivity to Touch : FM pain can be so sensitive that the weight of bed sheets or a light touch can be excruciating. Simple traumas like stubbing a toe or a bruise can be much more intense and last a lot longer in the FM patient.

3. Environmental Sensitivity : Things such as exposure to tobacco smoke, loud noise, chemical cleaners, and/or bright lights often intensify or bring on FM symptoms.

4. Muscle and Joint Stiffness can occur frequently, especially in the mornings and after prolonged sitting.

5. Muscle Spasms : Cramps, "Charlie horses," RLS (restless leg syndrome) are common, especially during the night, thus interfering with sleep.

6. Exhaustion : Sleep deprivation can lead to exhaustion and insomnia (lack of sleep) is a common FM issue. This can lead to chronic fatigue, causing energy levels to crash.

7. Concentration Problems : Brain or "cognitive" function is a frequent problem affecting short term memory, information retention, "mental fog", trouble concentrating/staying on task, and at times, dizziness.

8. Chronic Headaches : Tension and stiffness in the neck, shoulders, and upper back often results in tension and / or migraine headaches. Environmental triggers may be associated with the headache onset such as smells, light, or loud sounds (see #3).

9. Bowel Problems : FM and conditions like irritable bowel syndrome (IBS) often co-exist which can cause diarrhea and constipation, often changing back and forth. Here, a change in diet can be particularly helpful!

10. Depression : Like IBS, depression and FM are commonly matched and it often arises from having to deal with chronic, amplified pain, not being able to participate in family or social events, and low energy levels. This can be a "vicious cycle" as the more that activity interference occurs, the greater the risk/level of depression. This can lead to becoming afraid to walk, exercise, and getting out, which can feed the depression.

Obviously, there are many other signs and symptoms commonly associated with FM, but these seem almost "universal." Next month, we will look at ways to "beat" these 10 common complaints and offer some treatment solutions! Chiropractic care has been found to greatly facilitate FM sufferers and is an important player in managing the FM patient.

Fibromyalgia and Vitamin D Deficiency

Utilizing dietary approaches to help with fibromyalgia (FM) management has been our main topic these past two issues and serves as GREAT background information for this month's topic: Vitamin D and its role in the management of pain associated with FM. Let's take a look!

Vitamin D is found in foods such as fish, eggs, fortified milk, cod liver oil, and more. The sun also helps the body produce vitamin D with as little as 10 minutes of exposure reported to be enough to prevent deficiency. There are several different forms of vitamin D, of which two are important in humans: vitamin D2 (made by plants), and D3 (made by human skin exposed to sunlight). Foods may be fortified with either type, and supplements are available in both forms (D3 is preferred). The main role of vitamin D is to maintain normal blood levels of calcium and phosphorus. Calcium and vitamin D are often taken together to improve bone health and reduce fractures. Research has also shown that vitamin D may protect against osteoporosis, high blood pressure, cancer, and other diseases. "Classic" vitamin D deficiency diseases include bone softening conditions such as rickets (in children) and osteomalacia (in adults). People at high risk include the elderly, individuals who are obese, and those with limited sun exposure. Individuals with conditions such as cystic fibrosis (mucous build-up in the lungs) or inflammatory bowel disease are also at risk for vitamin D deficiency. With that background information, can vitamin D help FM patients with chronic pain?

In a February 2014 study (journal: Pain 2014, Feb 01;155(2)261-268), the first known randomized, placebo-controlled trial was conducted on 30 FM women with serum D3 levels below 32ng/mol/L (80nmol/L). Half were assigned to either vitamin D replacement or a control group that received a placebo (NOT vitamin D). The two groups were re-evaluated again after 24 weeks. The main hypothesis was that those treated with vitamin D3 would have less pain (as measured on a 0-100 pain scale and several additional questionnaires). The study found that there was a marked reduction in pain perception in the FM women treated with D3. Though a larger scale study was recommended to solidify these findings, the authors conclude, "This economical therapy with a low side effect profile may well be considered in patients with FMS." This study is important, as dosing of vitamin D3 (preferred over D2 commonly prescribed) was based on deficiency levels and provided at 1200 to 2400 IU/day. By the end of three months, those receiving D3 improved from an average of 20 ng/ml to almost 50 ng/ml and reported a 20 point decrease in pain on a 0-100 scale. Further, about 20-25 weeks after discontinuing D3, their levels dropped back to ~26 ng/ml with a corresponding increase in pain levels (by 30%).

WebMD reports similar chronic pain benefits with D3 replacement. In 2003, they reported that D3 deficiency is high "among all U.S. ages, races, and ethnic groups over the past two decades." They add that a then-recent study found that out of 150 chronic pain patients, 93% of them had "extremely low" D3 levels!

Fibromyalgia: Exercise is "Key"

Fibromyalgia (FM) is now considered a central nervous system (CNS) disorder rather than a musculoskeletal condition. FM is managed best from a balance of different approaches including chiropractic adjustments, soft tissue therapies, modalities, exercise, diet, supplementation, sticking to a schedule, taking naps, stress management, cognitive behavioral therapy, and more. Common symptoms of FM include chronic fatigue and mental fog. The focus this month is on exercise and the benefits of exercise as it relates to improving quality of life!

Recent research has been published about the benefits of walking – not just for the FM sufferer, but for EVERYONE! Dr. Marily Oppezzo, a Stanford University doctoral adjunct professor in educational psychology and Dr. Daniel Schwarz, a professor at Stanford, have published very convincing evidence that walking is not only physically good for the body, but it's also mentally good for the brain! In fact, they've discovered walking actually improves CREATIVITY ! The study found that walking either indoors on a treadmill or outdoors BOTH similarly boosted creative thinking in participants! Hence, for those stranded indoors during climactic weather, whether snowbound in Wisconsin or heat bound in Florida, equal benefit can be obtained from indoor walking, even if it's not as much fun as being outdoors! Though past research has shown that aerobic exercise generally protects long-term cognitive (brain) function, until this study, the benefits of walking when compared to sitting had not been considered as important. These authors point out that TWICE AS MANY creative responses were produced by subjects when they walked (whether on a treadmill facing a blank wall vs. walking outdoors in the fresh air) than when they sat from a prolonged period of time. This surprised the authors who thought thinking outdoors would easily be favored. They also found that these creative juices continued to flow when the person sat back down shortly after a walk! Now that we know that walking not only facilitates our bodies but also our brain, are there other exercises that can help the quality of life for the FM sufferer?

Dr. Lesley Arnold, a psychiatrist and FM expert at the Univesity of Cincinnati, College of Medicine in Ohio, recommends "a slow but steady pace" when starting a program, making sure that pain and fatigue are under control prior to introducing aerobic exercise. She recommends an initial assessment of the person's current fitness level and then starts patients at one to two levels below that level, gradually building up stamina to a goal of 20-30 minutes of moderate aerobic activity 5-6 days/week. Exercises that emphasize low-impact, high-aerobic output are the best, and water-based exercises really fit that ticket due to the buoyant nature of water. Running in water against or without a resisting current and simply swinging the arms and legs against the resistance of water are extremely effective. A study published in Arthritis Research & Therapy reported improved health-related quality of life in women with FM for those participating in water aerobics. The soothing benefits of warm water is a good starting point, and classes are often group-based, adding social benefits of camaraderie and motivation, which creates a fun experience that participants can look forward to. Since FM is a CNS vs. a muscle condition disorder, another "brain" stimulating exercise includes simply balancing. Depending on the age, agility, and comfort of the person, try adding balance-challenging exercising to the mix. A good program to try can be found here: http://beta.webmd.com/fitness-exercise/ss/slideshow-off-balance-core-moves

Fibromyalgia: Do I or Don't I Have It?

Fibromyalgia (FM) is one of the most common types of chronic pain disorders with an estimated five million sufferers in the United States alone. A "hallmark" of FM is the difficulty its sufferers have in describing their symptoms. When asked, "…what type of pain do you feel?," the response is often delivered with uncertainty such as, "…it's kind of achy but sometimes gripping…it makes me stop what I'm doing sometimes for only a second or two, but othertimes, I have to sit or lay down until it passes." It's sometimes referred to as "deep inside" or radiating, shooting, tender, pins and needles, and locating the pain is another big challenge. It's often a "generalized" deep ache that includes multiple body areas, sometimes all at once. At other times, it's spotty and moves around. It's typically NOT restricted to one side of the body but rather on both sides. It is these inconsistencies that makes diagnosing FM so challenging, sometimes to the point where it can literally take YEARS before a patient is diagnosed. One study reported that of the 92% FM sufferers who had discussed their complaints with a primary care doctor, only 24% lead to the diagnosis of FM! It is often asked what makes FM so difficult to diagnose and the answer is simply, "…we can't see it," and, there are no definitive diagnostics like a blood test, an x-ray, or

180

even more sophisticated tests that can be relied upon to easily make the diagnosis. Moreover, many FM sufferers have other conditions that overshadow FM signs and symptoms that often become the focus of her (or his) doctor.

Back in the early 1990s, the American College of Rheumatology reported "a system" for diagnosing FM. This consisted of a physical examination approach where a certain amount of pressure applied to at least 11 of 18 "tender points" had to be present. This was initially received with enthusiasm, as previously FM was a diagnosis made almost entirely on "gut instinct." However, it soon became apparent that it was not so easy to interpret the patient's response when these tender points were tested. Today, for a diagnosis to be made, there are three specific findings that are considered: 1) Wide spread muscle pain (in all four quadrants); 2) Pain that has been present for at least three months; and, 3) at least 11 of the 18 tender points are found – LESS emphasis is placed on the latter. The Fibromyalgia Pain Assessment Tool is a questionnaire filled out by the patient that can also help lead to the diagnosis of FM. Assessing the FM patient for other complaints or conditions commonly associated with FM include the following (% prevalence is reported by fibrocenter.com): 1) Irritable bowel syndrome (32-80%); 2) Temporomandibular disorder (TMD) (75%); 3) Chronic fatigue syndrome – sometimes to the point where bed rest is mandatory (21-80%); 4) Tension or migraine headaches (10-80%); 5) Multiple chemical toxicities; (35-55%); 6) Interstitial cystitis (21%) which includes ≥ eight months of bladder pain, urinary urgency, and frequency (more eight times a day and two times a night); 7) Restless leg syndrome (32%); and 8) Numbness, especially the hands and/or feet (44%). Other common complaints include sleep interference, which prevents deep sleep to be reached, depression or anxiety, concentration and/or memory problems, and more!

As chiropractors, we are trained to assess the FM patient, establish the diagnosis, and offer management strategies such as spinal manipulation, massage, exercise training, nutritional counciling, modalities, and more, which can significantly improve the quality of life of the FM patient. To achieve the best outcome, you may require the services of other types of healthcare providers, as the importance of co-management cannot be overemphasized!

Fibromyalgia "(More) Facts"

Fibromyalgia (FM) has been described as being a "myth" as well as "real" (and probably everything in between the two). This is a VERY controversial disorder that some doctors push under the rug by saying, "....there is no such thing," while others stake their reputation on it. So with this wide variance in attitude and beliefs about FM, what ARE the facts?

Fibromyalgia has been defined as "...a complex chronic pain disorder that affects an estimated 10 million Americans" by the National Fibromyalgia Association. FM mainly affects women but both men and children can develop the condition as well. Fibromyalgia can be subtle, hardly interfering with life and all of its activities to being totally disabling, disallowing participation in work and the most desired aspects of daily living.

DIAGNOSIS: In 1990, the American College of Rheumatology (ACR) introduced the diagnostic criteria for FM. This includes a patient's history of "wide spread pain" for at least three months, AND pain in 11 or more of the 18 specific tender points using 4 kg of pressure. Due to the significant controversy about the reality of the disease (as stated in the opening paragraph), ONLY a physician knowledgeable about FM should make the diagnosis. Along with this diagnostic responsibility, ALL other conditions having similar presenting symptoms as FM must be ruled out BEFORE making the diagnosis of FM.

SYMPTOMS: Though the hallmark of FM is widespread, generalized pain (in all four body quadrants), a number of other symptoms are common among FM sufferers. Some of these include fatigue (moderate to severe), sleep disorders, brain fog, irritable bowel syndrome (IBS), headaches (including migraine), anxiety, depression, and environmental sensitivities. Studies suggest that there is a "neuroendocrine" (nerves and hormones) abnormality that may contribute to FM symptoms.

CAUSES: Research has found a genetic link, as FM is OFTEN seen in several family members (among siblings and/or mothers and their children). "Secondary fibromyalgia" arises AFTER other health-related issues occur such as physical trauma (like an acute injury or illness), which can act as a "trigger" for initiating FM. Recently, more attention has been directed to the central nervous system as the "underlying mechanism" for developing FM. Here, the threshold or level of a stimulus that triggers a painful response is found to be much lower in FM patients compared to a healthy group of people (this is called "central sensitization"). Thus, a pain response is amplified in the FM patient due to this lowered threshold of pain tolerance.

TREATMENT: As there is NO KNOWN cure for FM, symptomatic support and functional improvement are two important primary goals when treating patients with the condition. In the medical world, there are MANY drugs that have been utilized for FM (such as sleep aids, muscle relaxers, anti-inflammatory, analgesics, and anti-depressants / -anxiety meds). ALTERNATIVE therapies include massage therapy, chiropractic, myofascial release, acupuncture, herbal supplements, yoga, and other exercise approaches such as swimming and/or simply walking are popular care options for many FM patients. Increasing rest, pacing daily activities (to avoid "over-use"), stress management, exercise, and nutritional support can ALL HELP reduce FM symptoms and improve quality of life!

Fibromyalgia – It's Hard to Explain!

Fibromyalgia (FM) is a condition that typically has a slow, gradual onset that starts out mild and gradually worsens. The symptoms associated with FM include generalized pain all over the body (above and below the waist including neck, shoulders, chest, upper back, arms, hips, buttocks, legs, and feet). The pain can be symmetrical or more intense on the left or right side AND it can vary from day to day. To top it all off, the pain is "chronic" and is usually present for three or more months, sometimes for years, before the FM patient might even mention it to their health care provider. The onset can be so gradual that other issues often become the center of focus until the intensity gets to the point where the patient FINALLY complains.

To better appreciate the complexity of FM, there are two types of FM: Primary and Secondary. Primary FM has no specific cause while secondary FM is linked to something such as trauma associated with a car accident or sports injury, a condition such as irritable bowel syndrome (IBS), chronic fatigue syndrome, restless leg syndrome (RLS), and others. Either way, it is often NOT the kind of thing many patients "bring up" during the discussion of history with their health care provider, especially if something else is bothering them that may be more pressing

So, how does one explain the symptoms of FM? Words such as a deep ache, burning, tingling, shooting, tender, pins and needles, stiffness, and flu-like symptoms are often utilized when describing FM symptoms. Almost always, these complaints have been present for a long time – or for at least three months. Often, the patient is reluctant and almost embarrassed to mention it due to the difficulty in describing the symptoms and the fact that they often don't know the cause. Equally, many doctors, "have an attitude" that is negative and/or non-supportive of the diagnosis of FM making it even more likely FM patients won't pursue the condition with other health care providers. This polarization by physicians is a very common issue and often the reason FM sufferers continue to "put up" with their condition rather than consult with others.

The KEY to the diagnosis of FM includes the following: 1) Widespread pain NOT limited to one area of the body; 2) Greater than three months of symptom duration; 3) Symptoms including fatigue, sleep disturbance, depression/anxiety, as well as memory and/or concentration complaints; 4) Symptoms severe enough that they interfere with daily living activities/daily life; and 5) Difficulty finding an answer to the cause of the symptoms, USUALLY involving more than one health care provider. Even though awareness by both the general population and health care providers has improved in the last few years, research has shown that 92% of FM patients have talked to their doctor about their complaints, but this resulted in only 24% being diagnosed.

Another challenge confronting healthcare providers in making a diagnosis of fibromyalgia is because it can't be seen on an x-ray or as an alteration on a blood test. Other diseases have to be "ruled out" before the diagnosis is even considered, but as was previously stated, secondary FM results from other conditions making it ALL the more challenging! It boils down to a very careful history and a physical exam has to be performed by the health care provider and the provider MUST believe in the diagnosis of FM. Tools such as the Fibromyalgia Pain Assessment can also be very helpful AND it's available online for the FM patient to access. Bring those results with you to the provider for added help in making the diagnosis!

Fibromyalgia Dietary Considerations

Fibromyalgia (FM) management from a multi-modal approach, which included dietary recommendations to reduce inflammation.

Anti-inflammatory foods can be broken down into four categories: 1) Fruits and vegetables; 2) Protein Sources; 3) Fats and Oils; and 4) Beverages.

In the fruits and vegetables category, whole fruits, berries, and vegetables in general are rich in good things like vitamins, minerals, fiber, anti-oxidants, and phytochemicals. In particular, green and brightly colored vegetables and whole foods (such as broccoli, chard, strawberries, blueberries, spinach, carrots, and squash) are great choices.

Besides being low in calories, high in fiber, rich in vitamin/minerals and more, berries EVEN taste good! For example, one cup of strawberries contains >100mg of vitamin C (similar to a cup of orange juice), which helps our immune system function. One cup of blueberries includes a little less vitamin C but it has minerals, phytochemicals, and anti-oxidants at only 83 calories per cup. A cup of cranberries has only 44 calories (it can also help with bladder infections), and a cup of raspberries has 64 calories and has vitamin C and potassium. Less common, but equally nutritious, are loganberries, currants, gooseberries, lingonberries, and bilberries. Put these, or a mixture of these, on salads, yogurt, or a whole grain cereal and enjoy a VERY satisfying snack or meal! The health benefits of phytochemicals and flavonoids include cancer prevention, bladder infection treatment, and may even help your eyesight (such as from lutein in blueberries and raspberries).

Protein sources include fish/seafood, especially oily ocean fish like salmon and tuna, as these are rich in omega-3 fatty acids. Soy and soy foods like tofu and tempeh as well as legumes are great plant sources of protein, though some doctors may recommend staying away from soy. Nuts such as walnuts, almonds, pecans, and Brazil nuts are also great protein sources.

Fats and Oils: Omega-3 fatty acids can be found in flax seeds, canola oil, and pumpkin seeds, as well as cold-water oily fish. Other fats that are anti-inflammatory include monounsaturated fatty acids, which are found in olive oil, avocados, and nuts and have been found to be cardiovascular disease "friendly" as well. Other healthy oils include rice bran oil, grape seed oil, and walnut oil.

Beverages: Our bodies need water! Of course, tap, sparkling, or bottled water are great sources of water. So are 100% juices, herbal tea, low-sodium vegetable juice, and if tolerated, low or non-fat milk.

Meal suggestions include: Breakfast – oatmeal with fresh berries and walnuts; Snacks – whole fruits, nuts, seeds, and fresh vegetables; Lunch and Dinner– choose fish and less fatty red meats; cook with olive and canola oil; load up a salad with fresh vegetables and fruit, avoid deep fried foods – rather, bake, broil, poach, or stir-fry instead. Fill up HALF of your dinner plate with dark green or brightly colored vegetables. Avoid the following: junk food, high-fat meats, sugar (sodas, pastries, candy, rich desserts, and sweetened cereals), highly processed foods, trans-fats and saturated fats (i.e., bacon and sausage), and white flour products (get 100% whole grain instead). Some research suggests not eating "nightshade plants" like tomatoes and eggplant.

Fibromyalgia Dietary Considerations #2

Fibromyalgia (FM) management must include dietary considerations, just ask ANY FM sufferer! Last month, we concentrated on the types of foods that reduce inflammation, but the question remains, what foods should we go out of our way to avoid? In other words, what should we NOT eat (and why)? Let's take a look!

As we all know, it's MUCH EASIER to simply grab a cookie, a chocolate bar, or go through the drive-through at McDonald's and eat on the fly. This has become "the rule" for many of us as we trim down our meal times to fit in other tasks. We seem to have our priorities mixed up and have become preoccupied in our busy lives using the excuse that "…eating simply takes too long."

The "avoid" list starts with stop eating junk food. It's like pollution to our body as it clogs and clutters up our digestive system and the absorbed by-products include "bad" fat like trans-fats & saturated fats that can damage the heart. These fats are found in highly processed foods, red meats, and high-fat processed meats like bacon and sausage. Many of these meats are also high in salt, another "no-no" for heart health reasons, particularly for those with high blood pressure. Other sources of saturated fat include lamb, pork, lard, butter, cream, whole milk, and high-fat cheese. Some plant sources of saturated fat include coconut oil, cocoa butter, palm oil, and palm kernel oil. The U.S. Department of Agriculture's 2005 Dietary Guidelines recommends that adults get 20-35% of their calories from fats. At a minimum, we need at least 10% of our calories from fat.

Other foods to avoid are white flour-based foods such as bread and pasta. This is primarily because white flour is derived from grains which are gluten rich (wheat, oats, barley, rye) and as we discussed last month, very inflammatory to our body! Simply avoiding gluten can be the nucleus of a great diet with benefits like increased energy, less mental fog, and weight loss without really trying! Sugar is also found in many products that we like eating. It's found in juices, soda, pastries, candy, most desserts, as well as pre-sweetened cereals. Even ketchup has sugar in it! Another "bad guy" comes from the nightshade family of plants that includes tomatoes, eggplant, potatoes (but NOT sweet potatoes), sweet and hot peppers, ground cherries (a small orange fruit similar to a tomato), and Goji berries. These plants contain a chemical alkaloid called solanine that triggers pain in some people.

Weight reduction is another way to reduce pain and inflammation. If your Body Mass Index is over 25, ("Google" a BMI calculator and check yours) then you may need to lose weight! There are MANY diets one can follow, but to keep it simple embrace one approach first and see what kind of results you get. Try the "Paleo diet" as it is a gluten-free approach. The Mediterranean diet is similar and then there is the Aitkin's Diet, the Zone Diet, etc., etc. Try eliminating the three most abused unhealthy foods in your diet (like soda, ice cream, chocolate, etc.) as that too can yield great results. Make sure your thyroid is working properly if you can't lose weight with these approaches. Simply put, foods high in sugar, saturated fat, and white flour cause overactivity of our immune system which can lead to joint and muscle pain, fatigue, and damage to blood vessels.

Eliminating these foods and eating the foods discussed last month is good for all of us, not JUST those suffering from fibromyalgia!

Fibromyalgia Diagnosis: A Breakthrough!

Confirming the diagnosis of fibromyalgia (FM) is challenging, as there are no blood tests to verify accuracy of the diagnosis like so many other disorders. However, blood tests are needed when FM is suspected to "rule in/out" something else that may be mimicking FM symptoms. Also, FM is often associated with other disorders that are diagnosed by blood testing, so it is still necessary to have that blood test. So what is the CURRENT recommendation for diagnosing FM?

The American College of Rheumatology (ACR) developed criteria for diagnosing FM in 1990 and has updated it since then. The original 1990 criteria included the following: 1) A history of widespread (whole body) pain for three months or more; and 2) The presence of pain at 11 or more of 18 tender points which are spread out over the body. The main criticism regarding this approach has come from the poor accuracy and/or improper methods of testing the 18 tender points. As a result, this examination portion of the two main criteria has been either skipped, performed wrong, or mis-interpreted. This left the diagnosis of FM to be made based on symptoms alone. Also, since 1990, other KEY symptoms of FM have been identified that had previously been ignored including fatigue, mental fog ("cognitive symptoms"), and the extent of the body pain complaints ("somatic symptoms").

As a result, it has been reported that the original 1990 approach was too strict and inaccurate because too many patients with FM were missed – 25% to be exact – by using this method. In 2010, the diagnostic approach was modified by using two different questionnaires: 1) The "Widespread Pain Index" or (WPI), which measures the number of painful body regions; and 2) the development of a "Symptom Severity" scale (SS). The MOST IMPORTANT FM diagnostic variables included the WPI score and scores of "cognitive symptoms," which includes the "brain fog" common with FM, unrefreshed sleep, fatigue, and the number of "somatic symptoms" (other complaints). The Symptom Severity scale (SS) incorporates these four categories and is scored by adding the totals from each category. By using both the WPI and the SS, they correctly classified 88.1% of FM cases out of a group of 829 previously diagnosed FM patients and non-FM controls!

What's important is that this NEW approach does NOT rely on the "old" physical exam requirement of finding at least 11 of 18 tender points. Because FM patients traditionally present with highly variable symptoms, removing the challenge of determining the diagnosis by physical examination is very important! Plus, now we can TRACK the outcomes of the FM patient to determine treatment success both during and after care. Since the 2010 approach has been released, it has been published in multiple languages and is starting to be used in primary care clinics. Recently, in July 2013, a study reported that the Modified ACR 2010 questionnaire is highly sensitive and specific for diagnosing FM, and its future use in primary care was encouraged. What is most exciting about this is that a referral to a rheumatologist may not be needed since this tool can be easily administered by primary care physicians, which include chiropractors!

In past health updates, we have discussed the need for a "team" of health care providers to best manage the FM patient. This multidisciplinary approach offers the FM patient multi-dimensional treatment strategies that encompass manual therapies, physical therapies, nutritional strategies, pharmacology, exercise, and stress management, cognitive management, and behavioral management. Now, with the release of the Modified ACR 2010 criteria, we can diagnose FM more accurately, track progress of the patient, and make timely modifications to the treatment plan when progress is not occurring. This is a "win-win" for the patient, providers/health care team, and the insurer!

Fibromyalgia and the Immune System

Fibromyalgia (FM) is a condition with a polarized audience comprised of those who believe it's real and those who don't. This interesting political-like conflict is, in a large part, centered around the topic we discussed last month concerning the causes of FM. This month's article will focus specifically on the immune system and its relationship to FM.

"EXTRA, EXTRA, READ ALL ABOUT IT! New research published on 12-17-12 in BMC Clinical Pathology describes cytokine abnormalities were found in FM patients when compared to healthy controls." OK! But what does that mean?

Very simply, this study reports that immune dysfunction is part of the cause of FM. The most exciting part is that this study identified a BLOOD TEST (finally!) that, "...demonstrates value as a FM diagnostic tool." Looking at this closer, the researchers used multiple methods to examine cytokine (proteins that help regulate our immune response) blood levels in FM patients. They found the FM group had, "…considerably lower cytokine concentration than the control group, which implies that cell-mediated immunity is impaired in fibromyalgia." This study's findings of an immune response abnormality strays from previous study findings which largely pointed to the central nervous system (CNS – brain & spinal cord) as the origin of the FM syndrome. This makes some sense as the study of immunology (in this case, "neuroimmunology" – the combination of neurology and immunology) has only been around for about 10 years, and as such, may hold some important answers as more evidence is uncovered to further support this potential "paradigm shift" in considering the primary cause of FM. The authors offer further excitement as this focus could lead to a better understanding of the cause of other neurological conditions such as multiple sclerosis (MS)! They go on by describing how body temperature, behavior, sleep, and mood can all be negatively affected by "pro-inflammatory cytokines" (PIC) which are released by certain types of activated white blood cells during infection. PIC have been found in the CNS in patients with brain injury, during viral and bacterial infections, and in other neurodegenerative processes (like MS)!

To further support this advance in understanding, the National Institutes of Health (NIH) reported, "…Despite the brain's status as an immune privileged site, an extensive bi-directional communication takes place between the nervous and the immune system in both health and disease." They describe multiple signaling pathways that exist between the brain and the immune system that function normally throughout our lifetime. When immune, physiological, and psychological "stressors" occur, cytokines and other immune molecules stimulate interactions within the endocrine (our hormone) system, nervous system and immune system. To prove this, brain cytokine levels go up following stress exposure and similarly go down when treatments are applied that alleviate stress. They list other conditions such as stroke, Parkinson's, Alzheimer's disease, MS, pain, and AIDS-associated dementia as being similarly affected as well. They also report that cytokines and other neuro-chemicals play a role in our neuro-development throughout our lifespan, help regulate brain development early in life and brain function throughout life, and how this all changes in the aging brain. There are also interactions of these immune chemicals that result in gender differences on brain function and behavior.

Needless to say, it will be very interesting to watch for additional developments along this line of research as it pertains to the FM patient and future treatment recommendations! Also, immune stimulation by chiropractic adjustments has been postulated as a benefit and this too may be better understood using this new research approach!

Fibromyalgia – Do We Know The Cause?

Fibromyalgia (FM) is a condition that is characterized by widespread pain, fatigue and an increased pain response. Symptoms can include tingling of the skin, muscle spasms, weakness in the arms and legs, nerve pain, muscle twitching, bowel disturbances, chronic sleep disturbances, and more. So, what can cause such a widespread, whole body condition? Though the "cause" of FM is unknown, several hypotheses have emerged. Here is what we know:

1. The brains of FM patients : Structural and functional differences have been identified in the brains of FM vs. healthy individuals. What is unclear is whether these identifiable brain changes cause the FM symptoms or are the result of an unknown cause. Some experts have reported that the abnormal brain findings may be the result of childhood stress, or prolonged, severe stress at any time in life. An area commonly affected is called the hippocampus, which plays a crucial role in maintaining cognitive functions, sleep regulation, and pain perception.
2. Lower pain threshold : Due to an increased reactivity of pain-sensitive nerve cells in the spinal cord and brain

(called "central sensitization), FM patients feel pain sooner and worse than non-FM subjects.
3. Genetic predisposition : It has been reported that FM is often found in multiple family members. This genetic propensity also includes other conditions that often co-exist in FM patients such as chronic fatigue syndrome, irritable bowel syndrome (IBS), and depression.
4. Stress & lifestyle : Stress by itself may be an important cause of FM. It is not uncommon to develop FM after suffering from post-traumatic stress disorder. An association between physical and sexual abuse both in childhood and adulthood has also been identified. Poor lifestyle issues including smoking, obesity, and lack of physical activity increase the risk of developing FM.
5. Dopamine dysfunction : Dopamine is a chemical needed for neurotransmission and plays a role in pain perception. It is also connected to the development of restless leg syndrome (RLS), which is a frequent complaint of FM patients. Medications found effective for RLS such as pramipexole (also used for the treatment of Parkinson's disease) can be helpful for some FM patients.
6. Abnormal serotonin metabolism : Another neurotransmitter, serotonin, regulates sleep patterns, mood, concentration, and pain and can be involved in causing FM. Decreases in other neurotransmitters (especially norepinephrine), when combined with serotonin depletion, can especially cause FM (more so in women than men). Hence, medications like duloxetine (Cympalta) originally used to treat depression and painful diabetic neuropathy, have been found to help FM patients, especially women.
7. Deficient growth hormone (GH) secretion : Abnormal levels of GH have been found in FM patients, but studies report mixed results when treating FM with GH.
8. Psychological factors : Strong evidence supports the association of FM and depression. Similarities include neuroendocrine abnormalities, psychological characteristics, physical symptoms and similar treatment benefits using the same approach (medication, counciling, etc.).

9. Physical Trauma : Trauma can increase the risk of FM. One report found a direct association with neck trauma and increased risk of developing FM.
10. Small bowel bacterial overgrowth : This can contribute to FM and may explain the association with IBS. The autoimmune response to the presence of bacteria resulting in FM symptoms has been hypothesized in these cases.

CONCLUSION: As previously stated, it is clear that a "team" of providers is needed to effectively treat FM. We'd be honored to be part of your team!

Fibromyalgia – Where Does the Pain Come From?

Fibromyalgia (FM) is a very strange condition. Can you think of any other condition that creates so many symptoms and yet all the blood and imaging tests are negative? FM symptoms include chronic fatigue, muscle aches and pains, depression, sleep disturbance, memory affects, and more. The degree or severity of FM varies from mild to severe, leaving some totally disabled and distraught. So, the question of the month is, where does the pain come from?

Since the usual markers of injury are negative (that is, blood and other tests), we can tell you first that the pain is NOT coming from damaged tissue such as muscle, bone, organs, and the like. If it did, abnormal enzymes &/or inflammatory tests would result. Rather, the origin of pain appears to be arising from within the central nervous system. That is to say, there are portions of the brain and spinal cord where pain signals are received and when they reach a certain level or threshold, the sensation is felt. When the sensory input is below that level, it will not be felt. In fact, there are MANY MORE incoming sensory signals that are NOT felt compared to those that are. This "thermostat-like" function is vital so we DO NOT feel everything that arrives to the brain. This is why we don't feel the clothes hanging from our backs or the shoes on our feet (unless the laces are tied too tight!). It's been said that if we DID "sense" all the incoming signals we would, in a sense, "…short circuit."

In the FM patient, this thermostat is "messed up." It is set lower than what is considered normal, and as a result, patients do sense or feel more than they should. This "nervous system overload," sometimes referred to as a "sensory storm," occurs in the FM sufferer. A more fancy term called "central sensitization" can be searched and you will find a LOT to read about this interesting subject (check it out)!

So how does this hypersensitive situation start? Fibromyalgia is classified into two main categories – type I and type II. In type I, or primary FM, the cause is unknown. The cause could include one's genetic make-up, but the bottom line is, we really don't know. In type II or, secondary FM, some other known condition or situation can be identified such as irritable bowel syndrome, rheumatoid arthritis, after a trauma, or following an illness or infection. Some also feel the lack of sleep or sleep loss can cause FM. This is because it takes about four hours of sustained sleep to reach deep sleep, and because of frequent sleep interruptions, the person never reaches deep sleep. Over time, deprived of the relaxing deep sleep benefits, the body gradually tightens up, "re-setting the thermostat" and too much sensory information reaches the brain, resulting in overload, and a heightened pain level is perceived. Studies have shown that when sleep is restored, many FM patients gradually improve and function better. This focus on sleep restoration is important in the management strategies of FM treatment. We all know our tolerance to just about everything suffers when we are over-tired, similar to the toddler who cries at the drop of a dime when they need a nap.

Chiropractic adjustments, certain nutrients like melatonin, valerian root, and vitamin B complex can facilitate sleep restoration. Treatment for sleep apnea can also help patients with FM. As we've said before, FM is usually multi-factorial and including chiropractic in the FM treatment "team" is essential for a satisfying result!

Fibromyalgia – How Aware Are YOU about FM?

Fibromyalgia (FM) has quite a history! There is evidence that dates as far back as Hippocrates in ancient Greece, when he described a mysterious condition affecting the muscles which portrays FM quite accurately!

FM is a complex condition that includes fatigue and chronic muscle, tendon, and ligament pain that is wide-spread (NOT contained to one small region). Generalized pain and fatigue are the hallmarks of FM, which can range from mild to severe disability. However, there are many misconceptions about FM.

How much do you THINK you know about FM? Try the self-test below. For each statement, decide if the statement is true or false. The answers can be found below...

FM shortens one's life span.

1. A patient may see several doctors before finding someone willing to help them.
2. FM can affect children, though it is most common in adults ages 20-55.
3. To properly diagnose FM, you must have at least 11 of 18 tender points.
4. With FM, you should not exercise if your body hurts.
5. A multi-discipline treatment approach usually works best (chiropractic, primary care, massage therapy, and others).
6. If you have FM, you were probably born with it.
7. Women usually develop FM more often than males.
8. The presence of pain associated FM signifies muscle deterioration.
9. It is easy to confuse FM with other diseases.

197

FM is present in 2-4% of the population and affects everyone differently, so each case is best managed by an individualized form of treatment. In other words, one treatment approach for every FM patient is NOT the proper approach. For some, fatigue is the primary issue, while for others, it's the sleep disturbance, irritable bowel syndrome. or bladder problems that require the most attention. There is frequently a co-existing psychological condition that may include depression, anxiety, and/or a stress-related condition, such as post-traumatic stress disorder. In reference to the 10 statements above, FM does NOT shorten one's life span, but it does affect quality of life. The primary goal of treatment is to help the FM patient gain control of their condition. It truly can take multple visits to different doctors before finding one that's willing to work with you and coordinate care with other "team" providers to give you the best quality care. FM can affect children, though it's rare – it's primarily the 20-55 year old age group with a 9:1 ratio favoring the female population. The "old" 11 of 18 tender point diagnostic requirement has been replaced by "widespread, generalized pain," NOT limited to specific points. Exercise is one of the BEST self-management strategies and should be encouraged. Though a genetic component has been identified, FM is NOT something you are "born with." The pain associated with FM is NOT indicative of muscle deterioration. FM is often confused with other diseases and the diagnosis is made by eliminating the other more easily diagnosable disorders. Chiropractic is a VERY important part of the management team in the care of the FM patient.

Answers: 1. False; 2. True; 3. True; 4. False; 5. False; 6. True; 7. False; 8. True; 9. False; 10. True.

Fibromyalgia and the Importance of Diet

Fibromyalgia (FM) management involves many treatment approaches. As was pointed out last month, the importance of sleep quality, hormonal balance, infection management, nutritional supplementation, exercise and more was discussed as the "SHINE" approach. This month, we are going to explore how important diet is in the management of FM.

It's been said that one of the most powerful tools the FM patient has in their possession is their FORK because, "…food becomes cells." That is to say, the food we eat is used to build cells, tissues, and support our organ systems. The National Fibromyalgia Association (NFA) has reported that all FM patients have some common physiological abnormalities that include:

- Too much Substance P (a pain producing neurotransmitter).
- Too little tryptophan (an essential amino acid that helps make serotonin which helps mood and many other things).
- Not enough serotonin (a brain neurotransmitter that fights depression)..
- Abnormalities in muscle cells, especially the mitochondria that provides energy (ATP) to the cell.

With the exception of substance P, we can control ALL of the above, at least in part, with diet and eating the right food. The following 7 nutritional recommendations can make a significant improvement for the FM sufferer:

1. ELIMINATE FOOD TRIGGERS: Eliminate foods that irritate the digestive system. The NFA reports that 40% of FM patients have irritable bowel problems and food sensitivities that trigger abdominal pain, diarrhea, and headaches. Common food triggers include: monosodium glutamate (MSG), caffeine, food coloring, chocolate, shrimp, dairy products, eggs, gluten, yeast, milk, soy, corn, citrus, sugar and aspartame. Regarding

aspartame and MSG - a 2010 study out of France reported FM symptoms subsided significantly after eliminating both from the diet, as they found that they stimulated certain neurotransmitters.

2. EAT MORE TURKEY! That's because turkey contains tryptophan, an essential amino acid that can help combat chronic fatigue and depression, which are common FM symptoms. In a large NFA 2007 survey of 2,596 FM patients, about 40% of the group complained of energy loss. Tryptophan is only acquired through food as our bodies cannot make it or convert it from other substances. Tryptophan is needed by our body to make serotonin (the "happiness hormone") which improves our mood and makes melatonin, the chemical that helps us sleep deeply. Hence, to fight fatigue, avoid the food triggers mentioned in #1 and increase tryptophan, which can be found in certain protein rich foods such as cold-water fish (salmon, tuna, anchovies, and mackerel), nuts and seeds, soy (soymilk, tofu, and soybeans), turkey, and yogurt. Many of these foods also contain tyrosine, which increases levels of brain neurotransmitters dopamine and norepinephrine. These brain neurotransmitters help with cell messaging, alertness, and reduce cognitive "fog," often described by FM sufferers. Also consider taking melatonin if sleep is an issue.

3. EAT MORE SARDINES! Okay, turkey is more "palatable," but sardines have the ability to reduce muscle pain, of which, according to the NFA survey, 63% of FM sufferers experience. This is thought to be due to coenzyme Q10 (CoQ10) deficiency, essential for muscle function and found in sardines and organ meats. Of course, if these natural food approaches don't appeal to you, a CoQ10 supplement may be easier. In two studies, FM patients were found to be 40% deficient in CoQ10, and 30% experienced less muscle pain and fatigue after taking 300mg/day for 9 months.

Stay tuned next month for the last 4 nutritional "tips."

Fibromyalgia and "SHINE"

Fibromyalgia (FM) management can be as difficult as making a definitive diagnosis. FM is characterized by generalized body aches and feeling exhausted, and yet, in spite of the exhaustion, the inability to sleep is a "classic" FM complaint. Some have referred to FM as "blowing a fuse" or as an "energy crisis," as more energy is expended than what's being made. FM sufferers, as well as the caregivers, know how physically and mentally difficult it is to manage this controversial condition. Many management strategies that have been published; SHINE is one approach. SHINE stands for Sleep, Hormones, Infections, Nutritional supplements, and Exercise. By focusing treatment strategies on these 5 areas, significant benefits can be achieved.

SLEEP: Some feel this is the most important problem to manage in order to gain control of FM. If we cannot reach "deep sleep," (which is the sleep stage that is usually reached after about the 4th hour into sleep) then the body cannot fully rest. When discussing sleep problems with the FM patient, it is common to hear them say, "...I wake up every 1-2 hours and can't get back to sleep for at least 15-30 minutes." This results in NEVER getting to the deep sleep stage and eventually, because the body hasn't fully relaxed often for years, everything starts hurting. This is the hallmark of FM. Some "tips" to help us get to sleep and stay sleeping include: keeping the bedroom cool (such as 65°), taking a hot bath before sleep to relax your tight muscles, spraying the pillow with lavender oil (helps promote sleep), taking 75-150mg of magnesium, avoiding caffeine (especially later in the day), the use of Valarian Root (a muscle relaxing herb) and/or melatonin (an amino acid that promotes sleep) can also help. The goal is to try to get 8-9 hours of sleep a night. Establish a routine in the evenings and go to bed at the same time or close to it.

HORMONES: These chemicals are produced by our endocrine glands (pituitary, thyroid, parathyroid, adrenals, ovaries/testes, and part of our pancreas. They are in balance with each other, and somehow, in FM they often fall out of balance. Have your health care provider perform tests (usually blood and/or urine) to determine your hormone levels and get them balanced!

INFECTION: The lack of sleep lowers our immune function, and infections can occur more readily. In addition to treatments, there are nutritionally based approaches to improve immune function, and if recurrent illnesses are part of your FM profile PLEASE consult with us regarding ways to boost your immune system!

NUTRITIONAL SUPPLEMENTS: This topic is related to the last as there are MANY supplement recommendations that have been found to boost immune function, increase energy, enhance sleep quality, and more. This is an area of FM management that is largely overlooked by traditional medical management approaches. Remember, a "team" of providers offers the FM sufferer the best way to manage this challenging to treat condition. Look for health care providers who are willing to work together as a team on your behalf.

EXERCISE: This is a MUST! For example, in a 2010 Oregon Health & Sciences University study, women with FM who practiced yoga for 8 weeks had a 24% pain reduction, 30% fatigue reduction, and 42% depression reduction.

Fibromyalgia and Neurotransmission

Neurotransmission is the method by which nerves "speak" to each other so impulses can be sent from one part of your body to the brain and back. For example, when you touch a hot plate by accident, it doesn't take long before you quickly let go of the plate. The reason you let go quickly is because of neurotransmission. Certain types of neurons or nerves (called afferents) bring information to the central nervous system where the information is processed and then signals are transferred back to the target site (such as your hand touching the hot plate) by different nerves (called efferents) telling you to immediately let go of that hot object. It's like the flow of traffic into a city during rush hour. People work all day and then drive in the opposite direction on their way home (afferents in the morning going in the city or "brain" and efferents in the evening bringing new information home). This "give and take" process of information coming in, being processed and going out helps coordinate our bodily functions. This allows us to constantly adapt to surrounding changes in temperature, stress, noise, and so on.

Each neuron has as many as 1500 connections from other neurons, but they don't actually touch one another. Rather, there are "synapses" where nerve impulses stimulate the release of calcium and neurotransmitters, which either inhibit or excite another neuron and each neuron may be connected to many other neurons. If the total excitatory stimuli are greater than the inhibitory stimuli, that neuron will "fire" and create a new connection resulting in an action (like dropping the hot plate).

Okay, sorry for the enthusiastic description and details of neurotransmission. More importantly, how does all this relate to fibromyalgia? A new study (published May 14, 2012 in NATURE by scientists at Weill Cornell Medical College) discovered that a single protein (alpha 2 delta), "…exerts a spigot-like function controlling the volume of neurotransmitters and other chemicals that flow between the synapses of brain neurons." This study shows how brain cells "talk to each other" through these synapses relaying feelings, thoughts, and actions and how this powerful protein plays a crucial role in regulating effective communication in the brain. They found that if they added or decreased this single protein (alpha 2 delta), then the speed of neurotransmission increased or decreased by opening or closing the calcium channels that trigger neurotransmission release.

The relationship between calcium and neurotransmission has been known for 50 years, but how to "turn on or off" the volume is a new discovery. They hope this finding will help in the design of new medications that will help regulate the neurotransmission in the brain, thus help reduce the increased pain perception found in people suffering from fibromyalgia.

Our aim in sharing this information with you is to keep you informed with what is on the cutting edge of research as we've said many times before, a "team" of health care provision is the BEST way to manage FM including chiropractic and primary care!

Fibromyalgia & Sleep

Last month, we focused on how important sleep is in the management of the fibromyalgia (FM) and the relationship between sleep dysfunction and Restless Leg Syndrome. Now that it's clear that the sleep and FM pairing is so important, how can we improve sleep quality? As stated last month, FM and sleep dysfunction go hand in hand and is a consistent complaint of the FM patient. The need to establish better "sleep hygiene" has been found to be one of the most important treatment strategies for those suffering from FM. This can help decrease pain, fatigue, and the "fibro fog" that is often described that impairs the ability to concentrate and work efficiently. Listed below are some sleep strategies that work very well, all you have to do is try them!

- SLEEP QUANTITY: The advice is to only sleep as much as is needed to feel refreshed and alert the following day. Getting too much sleep does not equate to good quality sleep. In fact, reducing the time in bed seems to improve the quality of sleep, as excessively long periods of time in bed result in fragmented, superficial or shallow sleep and doesn't allow one to enter the deeper, restoring stages of sleep.

KEEP A SLEEP LOG: Document the amount you sleep each night and pay attention to things that may have interfered with that night's sleep. You will find that reviewing these notes over several weeks will give you strong clues as to the triggers that interfere with your ability to sleep so you can develop strategies to deal effectively with these sleep barriers.

BE CONSISTENT: Establishing a regular time to wake up each morning as a consistent routine will help establish and strengthen your circadian rhythms, and a regular arousal time puts you on a consistent sleep cycle and leads to a regular time of sleep onset at night.

USE RELAXATION TECHNIQUES: The use of relaxation therapies such as visualization, deep breathing, a gentle massage, and southing background music or sounds are all great ways to boost restful sleep.

EXERCISE REGULARLY: This sounds counterintuitive but REALLY WORKS well! The KEY to exercise is to do this at least 3 hours prior to going to bed. Exercise not only "clears your head" but it provides a great way to reduce the accumulation of stress and exerts beneficial effects by promoting better, deeper sleep. Start slowly and gradually increase the duration and intensity of a form of exercise that you enjoy and look forward to doing. Pilates, Yoga, Ti Chi, Qui Gong, water aerobics, walking in the woods, or working out at your favorite gym or health club with some pals are some options.

BACKGROUND NOISE: Some FM sufferers really benefit from background "white" noise. Sound machines offer a variety of sounds that can help immensely! Avoiding sudden loud noises like low flying air craft or the slamming of a door or cupboard can disturb sleep quality even if we cannot remember the event the next morning.

NO NAPS PLEASE: Avoid a daytime nap; however, if you have to "recharge," keep the time short (no more than a 15-30 min. "power nap"). Long naps interfere with nighttime sleep.

TEMPERATURE: Keep your bedroom cool; warm temperatures interfere with sleep.

APPETITE: Consider a light snack rich in carbohydrates if hunger interferes with sleep.

NO CAFFEINE: Avoid caffeine or alcohol in the evenings as they both can interfere with sleep quality and the ability to get to sleep.

Fibromyalgia, Sleep and Restless Leg Syndrome

Fibromyalgia (FM) and sleep dysfunction seem to go hand in hand. In fact, most people who have FM complain of problems associated with sleeping. Sleep problems can include difficulty falling asleep with or without waking up one to multiple times a night. Also, the inability to reach "deep sleep" results in waking up un-restored. People with fibromyalgia frequently state, "... I feel exhausted when I wake up; I have no energy." They often feel more tired in the morning, and many go back to sleep during the day to ease their fatigue. Another common FM complaint is having great difficulty concentrating during the day, often referred to as, "...fibro fog." Other sleep disorders such as sleep apnea and restless leg syndrome are also often associated with FM.

Restless legs syndrome (RLS) is a neurologic disorder that is characterized by an overwhelming urge to move the legs at rest, thus interfering with sleep. Restless legs syndrome is more common among those who have fibromyalgia. Patients with RLS describe this as an unpleasant sensation in their legs and sometimes their arms or other parts of the body accompanied by the irresistible urge to move the legs in attempt to relieve the sensation. The terms, "itchy" or "pins and needles" or "creepy crawly" are frequently used when describing the sensations and can range from mild to intolerable. Symptoms are typically worse at rest, especially when lying or sitting and frequently results in sleep deprivation and stress. The intensity of the symptoms can vary, frequently worse in the nighttime, better in the morning. RLS may affect up to 10% of the population in the United States, especially women, and can affect both young and old, even young children. The severe cases usually affect the middle-aged or older and account for about 2-3% of the 10% incident rate. The diagnosis is often delayed, sometimes for 10-20 years. Although the cause is not clearly described, genetics seems to play a role given about 50% of those affected have a family member with the condition.

Other conditions often associated with RLS include iron deficiency, Parkinson's disease, kidney failure, iron deficiency, diabetes and peripheral neuropathy. Treatment applied to these conditions often indirectly helps RLS resulting in sleep quality improvement. Medications such as anti-nausea drugs, antipsychotic drugs, some anti-depressants, and cold/allergy medications that contain antihistamines can worsen symptoms. Pregnancy can also trigger RLS, especially in the last trimester. It commonly takes about 3-4 weeks for the symptoms to quiet down after delivery. Other factors that affect RLS include alcohol intake and sleep deprivation itself. Improving sleep and/or eliminating alcohol can be quite effective treatment strategies. There are no medical tests that confirm the diagnosis of RLS, but blood tests can at least rule out other conditions, and when all the tests are negative, the diagnosis is made based on a patient's symptoms, family history, medication use, the presence of an interrupted sleep pattern with daytime fatigue, and knowledge about the condition.

Treatment utilizing chiropractic management has been reported to be effective in managing RLS associated symptoms including the use of spinal manipulation, muscle release techniques, exercise training, and at times, physical therapy modalities. Nutritional approaches that emphasize muscle relaxation have also been reportedly helpful.

Fibromyalgia 101

Fibromyalgia (FM) is a disorder that includes widespread musculoskeletal pain along with fatigue, sleep disturbance, memory changes, mood changes, and more. Studies show that FM amplifies or increases painful sensations by changing the way the brain processes pain signals. FM is NOT a psychological disorder that only people with a troubled past or present acquire. Nor is it due to being inactive or lazy. If ANY doctor suggests that, PLEASE find a different doctor who understands the pathogenesis of FM. Unfortunately, this can be a challenge!

FM symptoms can begin after a physical trauma, surgery, an infection, and/or after a significant stress experience. It can also just gradually appear over time without an obvious triggering event. Women are more vulnerable to acquire FM than men. Many FM patients have other conditions that may be associated with FM including (but not limited to) headache, TMJ, irritable bowel syndrome, anxiety, depression, thyroid/hormonal imbalances, endometriosis, and more.

Though the cause of FM may not be clearly identified, studies suggest there are a variety of factors that work together resulting in FM. Some of these include genetics, infections, and physical and/or emotional trauma. Because FM tends to run in families, there may be certain genes or genetic mutations (changes that occur to genes) that make one more susceptible to developing FM. Infections appear to be a trigger for developing or aggravating FM. Post-traumatic stress disorder and less obvious physical or psychological trauma has been linked to the development of FM. The amplified or heightened pain response has been termed, "central sensitization," meaning, increased sensitivity to normal pain stimulation in the central nervous system (brain and spinal cord). Because of this heightened nervous system response, what normally isn't processed as pain in the non-FM person does reach and exceed the pain threshold in the FM patient (sort of like when amputation of a limb occurs and the brain still "thinks" there is a limb and "phantom pain" is felt). Studies show that repeated pain signals result in an abnormal increase in certain brain chemicals (called neurotransmitters). As a result, the brain's pain receptors seem to develop a "memory" of the pain and become "sensitized" or they overreact to the pain signal input and pain is felt at an increased intensity. Certain risk factors come into play with developing FM, some of which include: your sex (female), family history (increased risk if other family members have FM), and rheumatic diseases such as rheumatoid arthritis and lupus.

Tests to establish the diagnosis of FM are few. In 1990, the American College of Rheumatology established two criteria for diagnosing FM. The first is widespread pain lasting at least three months, and the second is the presence of at least 11 out of 18 positive tender points. Since then, less emphasis has been placed on the exact number of tender points, while ruling out other possible underlying conditions that might be causing the pain is now utilized. There is no lab test to confirm a diagnosis of FM, but blood tests including a complete blood count, an ESR, and thyroid function tests are commonly done to rule out other conditions that have similar symptoms. Treatment is best approached by a "team effort" combining the skills from multiple disciplines including a primary care doctor who "believes in FM" and is willing to work with chiropractors, and others. Exercising, pacing yourself, accepting your limitations, yoga, psychological counseling, nutritional counseling, and having strong family/friend support are all important in the management of FM.

What Causes Fibromyalgia?

Fibromyalgia (FM) is a chronic condition that impacts every aspect of life for those who harbor it. The diagnosis is often made on individuals with chronic widespread bodily pain in the absence of any specific condition and when no specific cause, such as tissue inflammation or damage, can be identified. Hence, the cause of FM remains illusive and confusing, resulting in beliefs that range from it being a purely a psychological condition to an entirely physical condition, while others simply do not feel it's a "real" condition at all. This begs the question: What causes fibromyalgia?

Thankfully, there is currently enough research published to confidently say that FM is at least partly (possibly mostly) due to a disorder of "central pain processing" (that is, how the brain "feels" pain), where a higher than normal pain response occurs to a normal, not-too-painful stimulus (technically called "hyperalgesia"), as well as a pain response that occurs to a non-painful or shouldn't hurt at all stimulus (technically called "allodynia"). There are several other conditions that include central or brain processing problems that include both genetic as well as environmental factors. Some of these include irritable bowel syndrome, TMJ or jaw dysfunction, chronic low back pain, and others. This central or brain problem may be caused by chemical changes in the brain which have been clearly identified in FM sufferers. Some of these include a deficiency (too little) of serotonin and noradrenergic substances, as well as too much or an excess amount of glutamate and substance P (chemicals that help transmit movement information from our feet and arms to the brain). In some cases, there are also psychological and behavioral issues that play a role in the cause of FM. Another study reported the cause of FM as being a "neurologic disease." They found that interactions of environmental stressors (financial, marital, etc.) PLUS "neuroendocrine dysfunction" (that is, hormonal and neurotransmitter issues) in people who are genetically predisposed to be the cause of FM.

So, it appears the
cause of FM is not one thing but rather, the presence of environmental
issues like stress AND chemical imbalances in our endocrine

(hormone)
and nervous (brain) systems that team up to clobber those of us who may
be genetically geared towards having FM. This explanation of causation
is important as there are both outside/environmental and inside/chemical
issues that MUST be addressed in the treatment or management program of
FM. This is why a "multidisciplinary approach" or a "team" of healthcare providers works so well in the management process. Because
there are biological, psychological, and social issues that require management, the team may consist of primary care (by a medical doctor
who is willing to work in a team approach and "believes" FM is real),
counseling, and chiropractic. Chiropractic is an integral, important
service to include as the primary complaint of FM is "widespread musculoskeletal pain" and NO OTHER profession focuses more on that
system than chiropractic. Patients with FM frequently report that a
regimented treatment plan that includes regular chiropractic adjustments, soft tissue therapies, often different forms of physical
therapy modalities such as electrical stimulation, ultrasound, pulsed
magnetic field, laser and/or light therapy, as well as nutritional counseling and exercise guidance are HUGE in the management process –
ALL of which can be quarterbacked by your chiropractor.

Fibromyalgia: What Resources are Available?

Fibromyalgia (FM) is a chronic condition that impacts its victims in every aspect of their lives. Many FM patients who present for treatment as their doctor about what resources are available for them and therefore, this is the subject of this month's article.

The National Fibromyalgia Association (NFA) was founded in 1997 in Orange, California and has become the largest nonprofit (501c3) FM-specific organization in the United States, if not the world. The initial goal of the NFA was to help patients with FM find doctors who were willing to treat and manage FM patients as this was a BIG CHALLENGE and remains an important focus of the organization today. The mission of the NFA is to improve the quality of life for the FM patient and to find a team who embraces that premise by creating and offering many programs, high profile media campaigns, and providing training to support group leaders across the country. Their philosophy is to, "…empower patients and to provide them with a new level of hope for the future." To that effect, the NFA evolved to include the development of an educational web site, the publication of an international magazine ("Fibromyalgia AWARE"), as well as developing medical education programs. The NFA website includes a "Resource" tab at the their homepage that leads to a listing of many great options that can be accessed at the click of a button:

http://www.fmaware.org/about-fibromyalgia/
Here is an interesting place for healthcare providers and patients with FM to review research articles on FM from 1981 to 2002, with over 300 references available:

http://www.myalgia.com/refs%2081%20to%200302.htm
Another good resource for information on FM is the New York Times Health Guide:

There are many places one can acquire information about FM. The list provided here barely scratches the surface. Simply google "fibromyalgia resources" to find almost anything you'll need.

Fibromyalgia: The Challenge of Treatment

Fibromyalgia (FM) is a disorder involving chronic pain that has no known cause. It is characterized by widespread musculoskeletal pain, sleep disturbance, fatigue and mood disorders. FM affects about 2% of the US population and ranges between 1% and 11% in other countries. It is more prevalent in adult women than men (3.4% vs. 0.5%) and is most common with increasing age with the highest occurrence between 60-79 years of age. The criteria for the diagnosis of FM was established in 1990 by the American College of Rheumatology as widespread pain of at least 3 month duration and pain on palpation (pushing with the fingers) of at least 11 of 18 specific tender sites on the body. Pain, fatigue and sleep disturbance are observed in all patients with FM. Additional features can include: stiffness, skin tenderness, post-exertional pain, irritable bowel syndrome, cognitive disturbances, overactive bladder syndrome or interstitial cystitis, tension or migraine headaches, dizziness, fluid retention, paresthesias (numbness), restless legs, Reynaud's phenomenon (white finger disease), and mood disturbances. FM is also strongly associated with anxiety, depression, chronic fatigue syndrome, myofascial pain syndrome, hypothyroidism, and many of the inflammatory arthritic diseases. Though there are no specific tests for FM, neurotransmitter deregulation including serotonin, norepinephrine, and substance P, result in an abnormal sensory processing in the brain and spinal cord. This results in a lower pain threshold commonly seen in FM.

The treatment of FM may be best looked at from 3 specific goals which include: 1. Alleviate pain; 2. Restore sleep; and 3. Improve physical function. Thus the most successful approach to the treatment of FM has been reported to be multidisciplinary or, involving several different types of health care providers. Clinical tools often used by doctors to monitor symptom change include a 0-10 pain scale, a body function scale called the Fibromyalgia Impact Questionnaire (FIQ) which measures physical function, common FM symptoms and general well-being; and, for measuring the physical and emotional side of FM, the SF-12 or SF-36 (SF = "short form" and either a 12 or a 36 item tool). The use of these tools helps monitor the success of the treatment that is being applied to the patient.

Though medications are reported as an important treatment option (such as an anti-inflammatory, analgesic, anticonvulsant, hypnotic, corticosteroids, opiates, various injections and more), the focus of this discussion is aimed at the alternative or complementary treatment approaches, as many FM patients cannot tolerate the side effects of the many different medications. Alternative approaches include cognitive behavioral therapy (counseling), exercise (strength & flexibility), acupuncture, and chiropractic treatment approaches, particularly manipulation but also soft tissue therapies and guided exercise training. Physiological therapeutic approaches frequently used in chiropractic clinics include low-power laser therapy, hydrotherapy such as whirlpool, Balneotherapy – using minerals and oils in the moving water, pulsed electromagnetic field, traction and massage therapy. Another exercise approach that can have great value in managing stress and facilitating sleep is Yoga. The key to a successful treatment outcome requires finding a "team" of health care providers that are willing to listen to the patient and work together to improve the patient's quality of life. Through this concerted team approach, in addition to the patient taking responsibility by performing exercises on a regular basis, following a proper diet, and getting adequate restful or restorative sleep, FM can be quite well "controllable" and, a relatively "normal" lifestyle can be enjoyed.

If you, a friend or family member requires care for FM, we sincerely appreciate the trust and confidence shown by choosing our services!

Fibromyalgia: The Challenges of Diagnosis

Fibromyalgia (FM) is a chronic condition where the diagnosis is made by elimination since there are no specific lab tests for diagnosis. In the past, we've discussed the different types of FM, the lack of good diagnostic tests, many management recommendations derived from interviews with FM patients, and more.

One of the many causes of FM involves the autoimmune system, thus suggesting that FM may be an autoimmune disease. In summary, the autoimmune system is very important system for all of us, as it controls the means by which our body fights off unwanted foreign particles like viruses, bacteria, and a host of other triggers that can negatively affect our body. The autoimmune process is best explained by example: Let's say a certain type of food is eaten to which a person has an allergy. As particles from that food are absorbed into the blood stream, the body senses that something is wrong –foreign particles are there that shouldn't be there. As a result, the body produces antibodies, which function like an army trained to "fight" the foreign particles. If the body's autoimmune system handles it without a problem, the person may not even know anything is "wrong" or that this process is going on. However, if the foreign particle is not handled easily or properly, then all kinds of symptoms can occur. In this food allergy example, stomach pain, nausea, cramping, diarrhea, and perhaps hives on the skin may even occur. Another common autoimmune example occurs in

215

the spring when flowers bloom, grass grows, trees bud, and so on. Many of us suffer from what is commonly referred to as "hay fever" and possible symptoms include a runny nose, itchy watery eyes, and sneezing (lots of it).

FM is sometimes thought to be associated with rheumatoid arthritis but the scientific evidence is not in full agreement with this theory either. More consistent evidence for causation seems to support the following possibilities: 1. Following trauma or injury. 2. A central nervous system origin (the topic of last month's FM article). 3. Changes in muscle metabolism. 4. A decrease in muscle blood flow.

However, there are still those who support the cause of FM being triggered by an infectious agent like a virus in susceptible people, even though no specific agent has yet to be identified. For those who state that FM is not an autoimmune disease, they do admit FM may have an "autoimmune component" to it. One study published in the Journal of Rheumatology reported, "…that scientists have discovered a new antibody in the blood of many FM patients." Subsequently, a new test was developed for detection of the "Anti-Polymer Antibody" (APA) that was reportedly found in more than 60% of FM patients with severe symptoms. The idea of a specific blood test for FM is certainly welcomed by all experts and clinicians who manage FM as a reported $16 billion/year in direct medical costs are associated with FM. Unfortunately, when comparing the APA levels in FM patients to those with rheumatoid arthritis and controls with neither, the APA levels were not able to distinguish between the groups. Unfortunately, until better testing methods are developed, doctors and researchers will continue to look for the "gold standard" FM test.

Fibromyalgia: "Why Won't The Pain Stop?"

Fibromyalgia (FM) is a chronic condition that does not limit itself to just one area but rather, it manifests as a generalized, whole body condition where basically, everything hurts. The diagnosis is typically made by exclusion or by eliminating all other possible conditions as there is no single blood test for FM and unless other conditions that are test sensitive are present at the same time, most tests come back negative. Of course, this leaves the FM patient upset because, "….no one can figure out what's wrong with me." We all seem to want a test to prove what we have is "real."

Unfortunately, in the real world, no blood test, x-ray, or exam procedure is 100% accurate (sensitive and specific), so even when tests return positive, there can be "false positives" that are caused by many things such as drug-induced test alterations and/or other conditions that alter the same test. On the other hand, there are "false negatives," so even though the test came back negative, it's still possible that the problem one is present but the test may just not be sensitive (accurate) enough to detect it. FM is one of those conditions where only after a myriad of tests have been run and come back negative, can the diagnosis of FM be made with some degree of confidence.

Essentially, we have to prove that you don't have something else causing similar symptoms before we can confidently (or at lease more confidently) diagnose you with fibromyalgia. To complicate this further, in "secondary FM," the cause of FM is known and is due to an underlying condition such as rheumatoid arthritis, lupus, hypothyroid, HIV, cancer, or a physical trauma such as a car accident or a work injury. When an accident is involved, the symptoms may be more confined to one area (then called "regional FM") making the diagnosis even more challenging as the classic 11 of 18 tender points may not hold up in these cases.

Finally, there are doctors out there that simply don't "believe in" the condition and may say to the FM patient, "…there is no such thing, it's all in your head. You simply have learn how to live with it. There's nothing that can be done." Well, they actually may be partially right – that is, the "…it's all in your head" part (don't get mad… just wait!). Another finding that is well-published in peer review literature is the concept called central and peripheral "sensitization." This occurs when increased incoming sensory information from injured skin, muscles, and/or organs "bombard" areas in the central nervous system (spinal cord and brain) leaving it "sensitized" or more sensitive to "normal" incoming information. This is because the threshold or tolerance to normal incoming sensory stimuli is reduced and results in increased muscle pain commonly described by patients with FM.

To better illustrate this, hypersensitivity or central sensitization has been observed in people following a whiplash injury. One study recruited 14 whiplash patients and 14 "normals" to compare their responses when stimulating the leg (the non-injured area) as well as the neck (the injured area). Theoretically, if central sensitization didn't exist, the responses to the exact same stimulus on the healthy leg of both the whiplash patients and the normal subjects would be equal. Instead, the researchers found the whiplash patients had significantly lower pain thresholds for 2 of 3 tests (a single electrical stimulus in the muscle, repeated electrical stimulation in the muscle and on the skin, but not from heat when applied to the skin). Each pain threshold was measured at the neck and leg before and after local anesthesia was applied to the painful, sore neck muscles. In the whiplash cases, a lower pain threshold was observed when the researchers stimulated both the skin and muscles at the healthy leg and at the injured anesthetized neck. That proves that the central nervous system has a "pain memory" which lowers the threshold so the whiplash patients feel pain more intensely and quicker than the non-injured people. This can help patients understand the answer to the question, "…why won't this pain go away?" This pain memory or hypersensitization is similarly found in FM patients.

Fibromyalgia and the Weather

Recently, a doctor had a patient tell him she had a "break-through" in her fibromyalgia (FM) symptoms that she was VERY excited to share. Having known this patient for a long time, he was intrigued by her enthusiasm. She told her doctor that her family had never had an air conditioner before until late last fall before the winter and hadn't used it yet until recently. She discovered that her generalized, whole body aches were significantly improved by running the AC, even when set at 79°F when the temperature outside may not have required it.

We all know that FM causes many symptoms such as relentless fatigue, muscle pain, depression, dizziness, nausea, etc. It's also no secret that FM symptoms vary considerably between seasons, as well as with certain weather changes, not to mention temperature changes, air pressure or barometric changes, and when it rains. As far back as 1981, a study reported that a large percentage of FM patients may be more sensitive to changes in weather compared to non-FM subjects. In fact, they stated 90% of the FM patients reported weather was one of the most important factors influencing their FM symptoms. Weather changes commonly influence symptoms in patients with other conditions such as rheumatoid arthritis, multiple sclerosis, and osteoarthritis. But, the question remains, how does weather affect fibromyalgia?

There are 5 major weather factors that appear to affect FM symptoms:

1. **Temperature:** Especially rapid changes in temperature and cold tend to irritate while warm temperatures are less troublesome.

2. **Barometric Pressure:** This is the measure of weight (pressure) that is exerted by the air that is all around us. Sunny days create a high barometric pressure while storms result in a sudden drop. These changes can trigger muscle aches in FM patients.
3. **Humidity:** This refers to the amount of water vapor present in air. Humidity is associated with headaches, stiffness, and widespread pain flare-ups in FM patients.
4. **Precipitation:** This refers to any type of water that falls from the sky to the ground (rain, sleet, snow, hail) and is usually associated with a change (usually a drop) in barometric pressure. This can result in increased pain and fatigue in FM patients
5. **Wind:** In general, wind usually causes a decrease in barometric pressure regardless of its force and therefore can trigger fatigue, headache, and muscle pain in FM patients.

Though a number of studies are available that support weather's adverse effects on the FM patient, researchers still are not exactly sure why this occurs but offer several explanations for this. One has to do with our sleep cycle. It appears that changes in the sleep cycle occur at times of extreme temperature – either hot or cold and this can negatively affect the FM patient. Another explanation involves the changes in our Circadian Rhythm that normally occurs with the changes in seasons due to the amount of light our body receives, less in the winter, more in the summer causing fatigue and achiness. The third explanation is the relationship between low temperature levels and an increase in the number of "pro-inflammatory cytokines" in the body, which increases pain intensity. FM patients have reported benefits from dressing in layers, avoiding cold temperatures, and increasing the amount of light inside the house (halogen bulbs or a light box, for example—taking Vitamin D can help too!).

We have discussed fibromyalgia (FM) from many perspectives but what we haven't done yet is listen to what actual FM patients have to say about what works and what doesn't work. Rather than reading about what "the experts" say about FM and what to do for it, let's take a different perspective – let's talk to those who have FM and hear what they have to say about the "do's and don'ts."

Consider the following great "pearls of wisdom" for those suffering from FM:

- Stick to a schedule—it helps.

- Know when you're pushing too much, and listen to what your body is telling you.

- Keep a journal every day about what you do and how you feel.

- Focus on the 4 P's: pacing, problem solving, prioritizing, and planning.

- Work on your communication skills, and don't be afraid to ask for what you need.

- Exercise and diet are very important.

- Acknowledge your limits—recognize what you can and cannot do.

- Exercise if you can—swimming helps me because it's easier on my joints.

- Don't overdo it or your symptoms will really kick in.

- Know your limitations—if you're tired, know when to rest.

- Join a support group—or even start one yourself.

- Stay informed—there's a lot of research and helpful information out there.

- Find a doctor who really sits down and listens to you and understands your pain.

- Use your friends and family as support.

- Learn about Fibromyalgia by reading up on the subject.

- Accept help when you need it.

- Wear a sweat suit when you exercise on the stationary bike; the heat may help to soothe your muscles.

- Sleep is very important. Try not to nap during the day so you can sleep better at night.

- Balance your meals with a low-fat, high-protein diet. Drink plenty of water.

- Stretching, swimming, walking, and a little yoga may help you deal with the pain.

- Keep moving and enjoy life.

- Exercise! Keep those muscles and bones flexed and firm. But do not overdo it!

- Write down the things that may have brought about your pain.

- Keep this list on your refrigerator as a reminder.

- This is just one way to help you manage the severity of your next "bad" day.

- List the people you can rely on ahead of time to help you on your "bad" days.

- Just knowing that you have backup may help reduce your stress.

- Your support network can help with completing important tasks.

- For example, on a "bad" day, ask them to run an errand or pick up your children from school.

- Sometimes, they could just be there to listen.

Fibromyalgia - More Tips From Patients

Last month, we listed many great "pearls" of wisdom direct from patients suffering with Fibromyalgia (FM), some of which we would like to directly focus on this month and expand as these truly arise from the heart of the experienced and deserve more attention (plus, we couldn't include them all last month and can expand on them now).

- **"Keep a journal every day about what you do and how you feel. "**Many times when discussing your symptoms of FM with your doctor, it is very hard to remember important details and keeping a journal is REALLY appreciated as it serves as a reminder for the patient of the things that trigger a flair-up. The journal can often save an immense amount of time trying to determine what can be done to help the patient, such as when to employ biofeedback skills, like visualization. This is performed any time or place where you may find yourself in a situation that is totally out of your control and you sense your ability to cope is failing. At uncontrolled times such as this, shutting the eyes and visualizing a calming and relaxing scenario is usually very helpful and can be exercised as often or for as long as needed. Again, write down the most effective visualization scenarios or thoughts so you can refresh your memory from time to time.

- **"Sleep is very important. Try not to nap during the day so you can sleep better at night."** One of the biggest complaints from FM patients is sleep disturbance, whether it's getting to sleep or waking up multiple times a night and/or not being able to return to sleep. Many "pearls" were found that dealt with sleep quality and methods for improving sleep. One of the most important issues is stated above – try to avoid napping during the day. Another is to go to sleep at the same time each night or to stay on a consistent schedule. Some recommended avoiding thoughts about the day that are stressful or situations you can't control prior to going to sleep.

- **"Exercise on a regular basis."** This too was a popular recommendation. Most felt "light exercises" was better, while a few favored strenuous exercises. Some gave specific recommendations like yoga, stretching, or swimming (".. because it's easier on my joints."). Some gave specific instructions like, "…Exercise! Keep those muscles and bones flexed and firm. But do not overdo it!" Another recommended wearing a sweat suit to keep the muscles warm. Most importantly, develop a routine that includes regular exercise doing something you like! This will ensure consistency and flow. Exercise also has the very important ability to reduce stress simply from "working out," and stress reduction and control was mentioned by itself multiple times. Not mentioned is the fact that endorphins and enkephlins are released with exercise that can reduce pain, as they are "natural pain killing" morphine-like substances our body produces.

- **Diet:** This too was popular and frequently mentioned. Some gave very detailed information about what to eat such as, "Balance your meals with a low-fat, high-protein diet. Drink plenty of water." A low-gluten diet is anti-inflammatory and very helpful.
- **Miscellaneous:** Educate yourself about FM by gathering as much information as possible, reading about FM on a regular basis, starting or attending a support group, and choosing a doctor who understands FM were also very common themes. Perhaps most important was, "accept your limitations," and in doing so, don't be afraid to ask for help – create a list of reliable friends and family who are willing to help out when needed.

Fibromyalgia - How To "Live With" FM

Fibromyalgia (FM) is a condition that produces widespread pain that can literally change the life of a FM patient, but as they say, "..life must go on!" Therefore, this article is dedicated to discussing ways to empower you with tips to make FM as least activity restricting as possible. Ways to gain self-control of FM include the following:

1. **Exercise:** There are two forms of exercise you should include in your self-management program. One is light aerobic exercises such as walking and/or water exercises with the objective to increase your heart rate. The other is strength training with a low-weight / high-repetition approach emphasizing the part of the exercise where you slowly release the weight back to the start position (the eccentric part of the exercise). Here is a list of tips from the National Fibromyalgia Association that should help:

- Start slow – don't overdo it the first few times you exercise. Post-exercise soreness is normal but it's exaggerated in the FM patient.

- Listen closely to your body's feedback! Increase the activity according to your tolerance – NOT TOO QUICKLY!

- Start with only a few minutes of gentle exercise and work your way up.

- Walking is a GREAT form of exercise. It can be done inside (in the winter, for example), outside, and/or in water (to reduce weight-bearing loads).

- Track your progress by keeping a log of what and how much you're doing. This can be accomplished by wearing a pedometer (that measures steps), a heart monitor (that measures pulse rate), and keep track of the distance and time, when possible. Make notes as to how you felt both during and after the exercise.

- Stretch before and after exercising.

- Keep your chiropractor informed and work as a "team" to advance your program.

2. **Sleep:** A poor sleep pattern is the "norm" for FM patients. The pain associated with FM usually interferes with sleeps, which leads to more pain followed by more sleep disturbance – it's a vicious cycle that needs to be broken. The National Sleep Foundation and others recommend the following steps to help us sleep:

- Stick to a sleep schedule. Go to bed at a similar time each night, even on weekends.

- Room temperature – keep it cool, not too warm!

- Avoid caffeine especially towards evenings (coffee, tea, soda, and/or chocolate).

- Avoid alcohol before bedtime as it can keep you awake.

- Exercise in the afternoon, NOT before bedtime.

- Nap as needed but ONLY briefly – like 20 min. max.!

- Be comfortable – wear soft pajamas and consider a white noise machine.

- Bedtime routine – consider reading, listening to soft music – whatever works for you! Once you find a routine that works, stick with it!

3. **Diet:** Talk to your chiropractor about food allergies, gluten sensitivity, diabetes, thyroid function, medication/vitamin use, and any other unique issues that pertain to you.

4. **Emotional control:** Engage your family, good friends, your healthcare providers, and consider FM support groups. Meditation, deep breathing, and visualization exercises as well as cognitive therapy can also be very effective.

Fibromyalgia: Vitamin Recommendations

Fibromyalgia (FM) can be characterized by pain that is widespread but not limited to a single anatomical area. This article will concentrate on a few specific vitamin recommendations with the understanding that a "good" diet such as one low in glutens (wheat, oats, barley, rye), rich in fruits, vegetables, and lean meats, with an emphasis of omega-3 rather than omega-6 fatty acids, can be highly effective in and of itself. More importantly, it doesn't make sense to abuse your diet and expect any vitamin recommendation to be highly effective. So the plea is, PLEASE practice a good "anti-inflammatory" diet, such as that briefly outlined above PLUS take the following vitamins:

- **Multivitamin/mineral:** This captures a little of everything and serves as a foundation (like the base of a pyramid) for more specific vitamin recommendations. In most cases, it is wise to skip iron as this is not usually a missing nutrient for most people and can be toxic for some. However, if iron has been recommended for you, feel free to include it.
- **Magnesium (Mg):** Magnesium is a missing nutrient as most foods do not include Mg and it is a vital nutrient in many of the pathways where proteins, fats, and carbohydrates are broken down in the body. Since it cannot be easily obtained through the diet, a supplement of Mg is wise.
- **Omega-3 fatty acids:** There must be a balance between the anti-inflammatory omega-3 and the pro-inflammatory omega-6 fatty acids. Most people consume far more omega-6 vs. omega-3 fatty acids (instead of the other way around) by eating fast food and potato chips, for example. There are long lists of omega-3- and omega-6-rich foods available on the internet – just "search" these and try to achieve a 3:1 omega-3 vs. omega-6 ratio. When choosing this supplement, many options will be available such as, "1000 mg of Fish Oil." But, take a careful look at the label to determine how many pearls/pills are recommended per day as this can vary quite a bit. There are two primary active ingredients abbreviated EPA and DHA that are the important part of "fish oil." Generally, about 1000 mg of each per day is ideal, which usually requires 3-4 pearls per day (which may mean 3-4000mg of "fish oil"—not "one-a-day").
- **Vitamin D:** Even if you don't read magazines or newspapers, you probably have heard some of the many wonderful things about vitamin D. It's also been reported as an anti-depressive and more effective for reversing the symptoms of SAD (Seasonal Affective Disorder) than stimulation using the correct type of light. It is a strong anti-inflammatory and hence, has a role in the

treatment of most diseases as most conditions include an inflammatory component. The FDA has recently raised the minimum recommended daily allowance from 400 IU to 2000 IU/day. It has been reported that 70% of people living in the sunbelt are vitamin D deficient since most of us avoid too much sun for skin cancer reasons.

- **CoQ10:** This is a very strong anti-oxidant and it's been highly recommended for anyone with any heart-related conditions. Anit-oxidants have MANY health benefits! Try 100 mcg/day.

Fibromyalgia: The Dirty Dozen

Fibromyalgia (FM) is a common chronic condition that affects millions of people around the world. The overview of the symptoms is widespread pain in the muscles accompanied by pain, fatigue, and "…just feeling wiped out!" Sleep deprivation is a common problem and some experts feel sleep loss for any reason—stress, past injury, current illness, etc.—can result in FM and restoring sleep is a key component to treatment. Here are 12 key points to consider to effectively "manage" or gain control of FM (as there is no "cure"):

1. **Keep Moving:** Exercise on a REGULAR BASIS. The presence of pain is NOT a reason to avoid exercise. Exercise is not only good for your muscles but it also helps improve the circulation, maintain bowel regularity, and reduce stress.
2. **Talk To Your Doctor:** Always discuss your fitness plans with your doctor! It's important to have a structured plan to follow and most importantly, START SLOWLY!
3. **"Learn" Your Limitations:** Around the house, at work and in the gym, learn what you can handle by slowly introducing new activities into your routine. Don't feel guilty about taking multiple breaks during your day!
4. **Remember to Stretch:** Gentle stretching can be very rewarding as it can improve flexibility, improve muscle tightness, and reduce pain. Stretching can be done at any time of the day and

also as a "warm up" and "cool down" before and after your exercise session.

5. **Make It Fun:** Choose exercises that appeal to you such as bicycling, swimming, or walking! Exercise in a location that is appealing such as walking in a park or in the woods. Take your dog for a walk. Try to achieve thirty minutes of movement-based exercise each day.

6. **Set Realistic Goals:** Don't try to run a marathon on your first day of exercise. You need to determine what you can handle by gradually introducing the activity. For example, start with a 5- or 10-minute walk and set a goal of 30 minutes by the end of the 1st or 2nd week. Then, work on speed or pace. Make sure the exercises you choose do not aggravate your condition further.

7. **Make Sleep a Priority:** Restless, non-restoring sleep is a common complaint of FM patients. Exercise can really help faulty sleep patterns. Set a sleep schedule. Go to bed and wake up at the same time each day. Also, talk to your doctor about nutritional options.

8. **Block Out Distractions:** Use ear plugs, "noise machines," or an eye mask to block out sleeping distractions.

9. **AVOID Caffeine:** Coffee, chocolate, or caffeine-rich soda can disrupt sleep patterns well into the night. Avoid these for at least four [4] hours before bedtime.

10. **Reduce Stress:** Just struggling with FM is stressful enough! Yoga, meditation, and deep breathing and relaxation exercises can be extremely helpful is reducing stress.

11. **Learn To Say No:** It's OK to say "no." We're all too busy but with FM, additional worries and stress really take their toll!

12. **Socialize Wisely:** Socialize with people who have a positive attitude – choose your friends wisely. Remember, the glass is always at least "half-full!"

Fibromyalgia (FM) is a chronic condition that affects multiple body systems and is not limited to any one aspect of health. Because of this, there is no ONE diet that works the same for all FM patients. Since most dietary guidelines that address FM are based on general healthy eating principles utilized for many conditions such as hypoglycemia, diabetes, food allergies, headaches, digestive disorders, and fatigue, let's review some of the most popular and successful dietary approaches that have been reported regarding FM.

Basic Guidelines:
- **Carbohydrates:** AVOID all refined carbs (white flour products). Eat whole grain bread, oatmeal, granola, and nuts. Avoid artificial sweeteners and limit sugar intake to a maximum of 40g/2000 calories. Eat roughly 14 grams of fiber per 1,000 calories consumed. Your total carb intake from all sources should be between 30-55% of your total calories.
- **Fats:** AVOID saturated fats (these clog up circulation and lead to inflammation and pain). That means <10% of total calories consumed, so limit or eliminate foods such as cheese, beef, milk, oils, ice cream, cakes, cookies, mayonnaise, margarine, chips, and chicken skin. Eat mono- and poly-unsaturated fats and include regular amounts of omega 3-fats. Eat < 300mg/day of cholesterol. Try to avoid ALL trans fats such as cakes, cookies, crackers, pies, bread, margarine, fried potatoes, chips, and shortening. Take omega 3 fatty acids like alpha-linolenic acid (ALA) as these help make other omega 3 fats like EPA and DHA, and are very helpful for the brain. ALA is found in flaxseed, linseed oil, or cod liver oil. Limit total fat intake to 20-35% of calories consumed.
- **Protein:** Go easy on red meat as they are high in saturated fat. Instead, eat more fish and vegetable protein (legumes and soybeans are great). When eating meat or poultry, remove all visible fat and skin before eating. Maintain protein at 20-40% of

total caloric intake. AVOID: processed meats, especially salt-cured, smoked, or nitrate-cured.

- **Fruits & Vegetables:** Whole fruits are superior to juices. Include blackberries, strawberries, raspberries, kiwis, peaches, mango, cantaloupe, melon, and apples. Some FM sufferers cannot tolerate citrus fruits but if you can, fruits like oranges and grapefruits are great. Vegetables are crucial. Good choices include carrots, squash, sweet potato, spinach, kale, collard greens, broccoli, cabbage, and Brussels sprouts. These foods reduce the risk of developing chronic diseases (diabetes, heart disease, stroke, and some cancers).
- **Dairy Products:** Choose reduced or fat-free varieties of cow or soy milk. This also applies to yogurt and cheese.
- **Healthy drinks:** Drink 8 glasses of water a day or diluted fruit juices, or herbal teas. Drinking water helps flush out toxins. Avoid coffee, tea, and alcohol as these increase fatigue, increase muscle pain, and interfere with normal sleeping patterns. Limit or eliminate alcohol.
- **Healthy Snacks:** Chopped vegetables, unsalted nuts, and/or seeds. AVOID ALL commercial snack foods (except salt-free air-popped popcorn) as these are high in trans fats & salt. Avoid chocolate and candy.
- **Junk Food:** Regular consumption of this is BAD for FM patients due to the high levels of fat, sodium, calories, and general lack of nutrition.
- **Artificial Sweeteners:** AVOID them! Examples: aspartame, NutraSweet, and saccharine.
- **MSG:** (monosodium glutamate (MSG) and Sodium (Salt) can aggravate FM!
- **QUANTITY:** Eat smaller light meals, especially in the evenings.

Fibromyalgia & Chiropractic Care

Do you wake up feeling tired, washed out, and dragged down? Do you have generalized pain throughout your body that doesn't seem to respond to anything you've tried? Do you wake up multiple times a night and fight to get back to sleep? These are classic symptoms of fibromyalgia (FM). However, when caught early and treated appropriately, FM can resolve or at least be controlled. Chiropractic care and management of FM is very effective and is becoming increasingly popular among FM sufferers. The goal of managing FM is to return you to a productive, enjoyable lifestyle allowing you to function and perform all of your desired activities.

Chiropractic care is the most popular and sought after form of alternative care or complementary medicine with half of American men and women utilizing chiropractic care during the previous five years. Of all the available healthcare options, few have been found to be as satisfying to their patients as chiropractic with 80% of those seeking chiropractic treatment reporting significant pain relief, better functioning, and an increased sense of well-being. Still, many ask questions such as "What is the science behind chiropractic?" and "What exactly does a chiropractor do?"

The original hypothesis or theory of chiropractic that led to its founding in 1895 is that skeletal or bone misalignments cause nerve interference resulting in pain, loss of function, and a host of other symptoms related to the nervous system. The entire body is connected through bones, joints, muscles, ligaments, tendons, with their supporting circulatory or blood flow system and nervous system. When the skeletal structure is in good alignment, the body can handle the many stresses and challenges we all face on a daily basis. When there is a breakdown in this system, symptoms manifest and when left untreated, these symptoms can develop into chronic pain, including conditions such as fibromyalgia. Chiropractors focus on reducing pain and associated symptoms by correcting the imbalances in the skeletal system with the objective of reducing nervous system dysfunction. Many of the techniques utilized in chiropractic care include manipulation of not only the bony structures, but also the muscles, tendons, and ligaments through various forms of manual or hands-on therapy, stretching, posture correction methods, exercise, lifestyle modification recommendations including diet and nutritional management, and activity modifications. Chiropractic care also includes discussions and instructions for modifying methods of performing tasks including bending, lifting, pulling, pushing in both at work and home activities. Workstation modifications are also thoroughly investigated, especially when symptoms are consistently worse after the work day.

Patients with fibromyalgia classically have generalized pain and tender spots throughout their body and often present with back pain, neck pain, headaches, as well as arm and/or leg pain. Chiropractic care can effectively reduce the pain associated with FM by reducing bony misalignments, restoring muscle tone, and improving posture. Proper exercise training has been found to be very important in maintaining long-term control of FM and is included in the management of FM. Diet and nutritional counseling may also be beneficial. Research has been very supportive of chiropractic care for patients suffering from FM.

Fibromyalgia – Important "Fibro Facts"

So you think you may suffer from Fibromyalgia (FM) and you're trying to find out more information about FM.....but where do you start? Certainly you can "Google" the word "fibromyalgia" and spend the rest of the day, week, or maybe month reading about the symptoms, clinical signs, the many treatment options and the different types of doctors who treat FM patients. You will certainly learn a lot! But you will still most likely remain confused as to what to do about it.

First, what is fibromyalgia? It is a chronic (long standing) painful condition resulting in widespread pain throughout the body and it's usually difficult to isolate a cause or reason for such significantly disabling symptoms. It is very common, affecting 3-

233

6% of the general population (global) and 6-12 million Americans (2-4% of the US population). Woman are affected more than men (75-90% are women), and it is typically diagnosed between 20-50 years of age. It affects people physically, emotionally, and socially. The symptoms can fluctuate but it never completely disappears. The cause, though still debated, points to the central nervous system in which a "minor" pain signal reaching the brain is somehow magnified and perceived as more intense (this is called "central sensitization"). This makes the FM patient hypersensitive to normal stimulations like a hug or a when hitting a bump in the road with the car.

How is it diagnosed? Prior to 1987, it was not recognized by the AMA as an illness or cause of disability. In 1990, The American College of Rheumatology (ACR) reported the initial criteria for diagnosing FM. There are no blood tests, x-rays, biopsies, EEG's, EMG's or other tests for FM. Hence, a thorough history (frequently revealing fatigue, sleep problems, mental fog, depression, headache, and bowel problems) and examination ruling out other disorders is appropriate. Diagnosis includes a history of widespread, chronic pain and the presence of multiple tender points (at least 11 of 18) located all over the body.

What is the treatment? Pain management has been the focus and this can include medication, ice/heat, exercise, lifestyle adjustments, counseling when anxiety/depression are issues, dietary strategies, sleep management, but perhaps most important is education – about FM and how to "live with it." That is, learning how to "control it" since no one has found the "cure." Exercise in short durations of time by walking or swimming (not too strenuous). Expect post-exercise soreness so don't overdo it initially, or you'll be "convinced" you shouldn't be exercising. Diet – avoid glutens/grains and emphasize fruits, vegetables, lean meats (grass fed chicken, beef, and fish), and consider nutritional support from a multiple vitamin, calcium/magnesium, fish oil (omega 3 fatty acids), Vit D3, and Co-Q10. Find a good "team" of doctors – chiropractic, family doc, and rheumatologist who YOU are comfortable with and who will work together for you. Don't expect miracles – it may lead to disappointment.

Fibromyalgia – Coping Strategies, "What Can I Do?"

Fibromyalgia (FM) is one of the most common conditions associated with chronic pain affecting up to 5% of the population. It is characterized by pain in the muscles and joints and is associated with generalized, whole body muscle stiffness, body aches, sleep disruption, and headache. Stress is often a component of FM. Women are 2-3 times more likely to suffer from FM.

So the question is raised, "what can I do to reduce the pain and suffering that I feel from FM?" The answer is multifactorial as there are many treatment approaches reported to be helpful. Perhaps the most prevalent is exercise. This seems logical as often, the presence of pain is misinterpreted as a reason to rest or reduce activity. This inappropriate thought leads to de-conditioning or weakening of muscles, stiffness in joints, lowered aerobic capacity and a host of negative physical and mental effects that can have negative effects on quality of life. Because many patients with FM are "out of shape," the worst approach with exercise is jumping into it too quickly. The post-exercise soreness when people first engage in a new activity can be profound if the introduction into exercise is too vigorous, and again, the pain intensity may be misinterpreted as a reason to discontinue any and all future exercise programs.

Therefore, the key to success is realizing pain thresholds are reached faster in the FM patient and hence, a slow but steady introduction into exercising is needed.

For example, start out with a walking program of 5 minutes, 1-3 times a day, and gradually increase it to 10, 15, 20 and eventually, 30 or more minutes per session. Stretching exercises of the overly tight postural muscles like the hamstrings, calf muscles, hip flexors, lower, middle, and upper back muscles are very helpful. Applying light resistance during the stretch using a "slow motion" approach improves results.

In general, low-impact activities like water exercise, swimming, bicycling, and elliptical (low setting) are great options. Using light dumbbells/hand weights emphasizing high rep/low weight is also very effective.

Another highly successful type of exercise are balance stimulating exercises. That is, using a rocker board, wobble board, gym ball, and/or foam pad to incorporate balance challenges into the exercise process is very effective. Consistent exercise is a key to success.

Also, don't set your goals too high as you may be setting yourself up for disappointment. Rather, make realistic goals and "grow" with the exercise process, changing and modifying goals on a monthly or quarterly basis.

Posttraumatic Fibromyalgia

Fibromyalgia (FM) has a long reputation for being a controversial diagnosis. Some healthcare providers (HCPs) feel FM is a legitimate condition that warrants treatment and research while others feel it's a "garbage can diagnosis" that HCPs throw patients into when they're not sure what diagnostic label to use to describe a patient's condition. Regardless of the personal beliefs of individual HCPs, there have been two general classifications of FM: primary and secondary. Primary FM occurs when there is no underlying health condition participating in the patient's overall health status and the onset of FM. Secondary FM results from an underlying condition that contributes

236

significantly to the patient's health status, such as irritable bowel syndrome and over time, gives rise to the onset of FM.

Posttraumatic FM belongs to the secondary FM classification when the trauma-related injury results in the patient developing FM. A Canadian study reported that 25-50% of FM patients reported a traumatic event just before their FM symptoms began. This study surveyed different specialty physician groups to determine which issues were most important in causing the onset of widespread chronic pain after a motor vehicle trauma. Five factors were studied to determine how important each was to the HCP in arriving at a FM diagnosis in a case study of a 45-year-old female with a whiplash injury who developed chronic generalized pain, fatigue, difficulties in sleeping, and diffuse muscle tenderness. These five factors included:

1. The number of FM cases diagnosed weekly by the HCP.

2. The patient's gender.

3. The force of the initial impact.

4. The patient's psychiatric history before the trauma.

5. The initial injury severity.

The researchers also considered the patient's pre-injury health status, fitness level, and psychological health to be important as well. All HCP groups were reluctant to blame the car accident as causing FM, but rather placed more importance on the patient attitude, personality, and level of emotional stress. The least important of the five points were numbers 3 and 5. The orthopedic group also included "ongoing litigation" as a cause but as a group, they were the least likely to agree on the FM diagnosis (29%) in this particular case study. Rheumatologists were the most likely to diagnose FM at 83%, followed by general practitioners at 71%, and physiatrists at 60%. A most interesting observation was that once the data was analyzed, ONLY the patient's pre-accident psychiatric history remained in the model of predicting agreement or disagreement with the FM diagnosis.

Posttraumatic FM can result from any type of trauma, not just motor vehicle collisions. Other "secondary" FM causes besides trauma can include systemic conditions such as irritable bowel syndrome, chronic fatigue syndrome, and other internal disorders that in part, alter the person's ability to obtain restorative sleep. Hence, an important focus of treatment should be placed on helping the FM patient obtain restful sleep. Chiropractic management strategies have included manipulation, mobilization, soft tissue therapies, physiological therapeutic agents such as electrical stimulation, ultrasound, the training for home use of traction, the use of nutritional counseling and supplementation, and exercise training. Many studies support success with this multidimensional approach to treating FM as chiropractic attacks the FM condition from multiple directions, often yielding highly satisfying results.

What Is Fibromyalgia and Can Doctors Agree On the Diagnosis?

Fibromyalgia (FM) has long been considered a condition involving the soft tissues of the body, that is, the muscles, ligaments, tendons and fascia. It is defined as "a chronic, generalized pain condition associated with symptoms of fatigue, stiffness, and sleep disturbance and is characterized by the physical findings of local tenderness in many specific but widely dispersed sites. Fibromyalgia is the most common cause of widespread pain. The prevalence of this disorder in the general population is between 3% and 5%... Most patients with fibromyalgia remain symptomatic for several years, and no cure has been identified." Disturbances in the central nervous system (CNS) has also been linked to this condition.

In one study, 168 FM patients had the CNS evaluated by hearing tests, eye movement tests, and a test that evaluates balance/dizziness. Abnormal findings were common in the FM patient group compared to non-FM subjects. Another study utilized an electrical current treatment approach through the skull to stimulate the brain that was stimulated resulted in reductions of pain that lasted for three weeks and mild improvements in quality of life were reported.

Comparing 287 general practitioners (GPs), 160 orthopedists, 160 physiatrists, and 160 rheumatologists, evaluating a patient injured in a motor vehicle crash, those most likely to diagnose FM were rheumatologists (83%) with physiatrists and GPs in the middle at 60% and 71%, respectively. Orthopedists were least likely at 29%. There were five factors found to be important in the respondent's agreement or disagreement with the FM diagnosis:

1. The number of FM cases diagnosed weekly by the respondent (strong predictor).
2. The patient's gender (females > males was a strong predictor).
3. The force of the initial impact (least important).
4. The patient's psychiatric history before the trauma (more important).
5. The initial injury severity (least important).

This information is important as the shift from considering FM to be strictly a condition of the muscles and other soft tissues to being a condition of the central nervous system will affect our future treatment strategies. Obtaining multiple opinions from various types of practitioners will most likely result in a variety of opinions. **Previous reports of treatment benefit utilizing chiropractic approaches, exercise, and strategies to facilitate sleep restoration remain strong in the management process of FM.**

Fibromyalgia (FM) is a chronic condition characterized by widespread pain and tenderness in the musculoskeletal system. Patients with FM suffer from a multitude of complaints that may include not only widespread muscle aches and pains but also complaints such as those related to the digestive system (stomach complaints, bowel problems, etc.). There are many treatment approaches available for joint and soft tissue management but few have looked at the long-term benefits.

One study included both the short and the long term effects using connective tissue manipulation and the combination of ultrasound (US) with high-voltage electrical stimulation. The level of pain, the degree of restorative sleep, and the impact FM has on functional activities using a 0-10 scale, were followed with 20 female patients diagnosed with FM. Treatments included 20 sessions of daily soft tissue manipulation (muscles, joint capsules, and other connective tissues) applied to the back region. The combined US therapy was applied to the upper back region, every other session. The benefit of the treatment was evaluated initially, after the 20 sessions, and again after one year. All three issues tested (pain intensity, impact on functional activities, and complaint of non-restorative sleep) improved and remained improved at the end of 1-year. The benefits from the treatment lasted, at minimum, 3 months and 21% of the participants (3 subjects) were still pain free after 1 year. None of the follow-up subjects obtained additional medical and/or manipulative treatment though 5 (36%) began to use medications during that time period while 64% did not require any medications. Patient satisfaction using the 0-10 scale was high, reported at 7.14 (10 = highest satisfaction).

Another study utilized 15 subjects with 30 treatments, ¬performed at a 2-3x/wk frequency, of ischemic compression and spinal manipulation. The ischemic compression included thumb pressure applied to each tender point for 10 seconds applying progressively greater pressure up to patient tolerance. This was repeated until the point was no longer tender using 4kg of force or, the trial ended, whichever occurred first. Spinal adjustments were applied to the neck and mid back area of the spine. Three methods of measuring clinical change (pain intensity, sleep quality, and fatigue) were utilized at the initial, 15th and after the 30th treatment. A minimum of 50% improvement in score was required to be considered a good respondent. After 30 treatments, 9 were considered good respondents, while 6 were not. In the respondent group, the percent change/improvement was 77.1% in pain, 63.5% in quality of sleep, and 74.8% improvement in fatigue. At a 1-month follow-up, continued pain reduction was reported, unlike a similar trail testing the benefits of two popular medications (amityiptyline and cyclobenzaprine).

Of interest, many of the non-respondents were older, had a more chronic/long term illness, and had a greater intensity of symptoms with greater number of tender points at the start of the study.

Fibromyalgia And Your Upper Neck

How can a spinal problem possibly contribute to your fibromyalgia symptoms, such as chronic musculoskeletal pain? In many disorders involving musculoskeletal pain, the nervous system is involved in some degree and the nervous system itself can get affected by structural changes in the spinal column.

When viewing the neck from the side, there should be a forward curve with your head above your shoulders, not in front of them. When forward head carriage is present or when there is a reduction in this forward arch, this may cause additional strain to the upper cervical spine or spinal cord, potentially compromising the function of those delicate nerves.

241

The upper neck can also be influenced by a spinal joint dysfunction of the upper vertebrae, such as the atlas. This small bone supports the weight of the skull and is necessary for the great rotational range of motion of the neck. The atlas surrounds the spinal cord and as it displaces, it can also pull or tether the spinal cord, which may irritate the nervous system.

During neck trauma, the head and neck can be put through a violent range of motion that causes the soft tissues (muscles and ligaments) to tear. Blows to the head, injuries sustained during childhood or while playing sports, and even poor sleeping posture can cause the upper neck vertebrae to displace, injuring the soft tissues of the joint. Scar tissue can develop after trauma, which may affect the precise movements of the upper neck. Swelling and inflammation in the tissues near the spine can also affect the nervous system.

The disorders of poor posture and displaced vertebrae can be assessed through x-rays. Range of motion tests are necessary to see how your function may be affected. In some patients, fibromyalgia symptoms can improve substantially following treatments to address these sorts of issues. However, most fibromyalgia patients will need a comprehensive approach that also incorporates an exercise program and nutritional or weight loss support. Chiropractic care is a natural alternative for those who wish a drug-free and non-invasive approach. It carries few risks of side effects and is balanced by the potential to help patients who also have spinal disorders contributing to their poor health.

Depressed with Fibromyalgia?

Many patients with fibromyalgia have long-standing depression, which is more substantial than just having the occasional morning blues. Their muscle pain can either be a cause for their depression or even the effect of a prolonged, depressed state of mind. Or the two may not be linked at all and simply co-exist at the same time. In some patients, depression may lead to inactivity, an unhealthy diet and weight gain, or even substance abuse. These habits will generally aggravate fibromyalgia-related pains.

In addition to using chiropractic care to improve spinal function and posture, there are other important aspects to be considered when treating the fibromyalgia patient. If depression seems to predate their muscle pains, then a through work-up and perhaps counseling with a clinical psychologist may be of help.

Other patients can benefit from increasing their activity and starting a rigorous exercise program. Both strength training and aerobic activities have been shown in studies to help patients. For those with muscle pain, it may not seem correct to work the muscles more, but research has shown that increasing muscle strength can decrease pain in the long run.

Some people find exercise causes joint pain in their spine and/or hips. Exercising while in pain is no fun at all and cannot be sustained. This is where chiropractic can be an important adjunct to keep you moving.

Vigorous exercise can also raise endorphin levels, blocking pain and elevating your mood. In fact, several studies have shown that engaging in regular physical exercise can reduce symptoms associated with anxiety and depression.

A comprehensive approach is the solution to treating fibromyalgia. For some patients, medications can be life-savors. For others, the side effects will eclipse any benefits. More holistic approaches such as chiropractic care should at least be considered, especially if allopathic care doesn't seem to work for you.

Understanding Fibromyalgia and Your Options for Care

Worldwide, fibromyalgia affects up to 5% of the population or about 15 million people in the United States alone. Fibromyalgia is not a disease in the sense that it has a known viral or bacterial cause. Rather, it is a collection of symptoms, mostly pain, that affect the neuromusculoskeletal system. Since other types of diseases can cause widespread pain, these need to ruled out before a fibromyalgia diagnosis is made. In addition to pain, fibromyalgia sufferers may experience sleep deprivation (including lack of restorative sleep), general fatigue, and even depression. They may also have difficulties with concentration and even memory loss. Up to 40% of fibromyalgia patients are thought to have a mood disorder, such as depression or anxiety.

In terms of medical treatment options, there are antidepressants, muscle relaxants, anti-inflammatory drugs, and pain or narcotic medications. When the fibromyalgia patient considers these or any treatments, her or she should consult with their doctor as to whether the risks associated with such approaches are outweighed by any potential benefits.

Many patents do not consider non-drug treatments such as exercise and chiropractic care, but these less-invasive treatments are an important option.

Fibromyalgia patients with central (spine) pain may respond well to spinal manipulation and other forms of care offered at chiropractic clinics.

Though is seems counterintuitive, for patients with muscle pain, simply avoiding movement may worsen their condition. In fact, aerobic exercise (as well as strength training) can dramatically reduce muscle pain. Many patients also find their mood is elevated when exercise becomes a part of the daily routine. Additionally, sleep may also be more restorative when you use your body more intensely during the day.

Lastly, weight-loss and proper nutrition are essential elements to overall good health. The important thing to consider is a multifactorial approach, which addresses your weight and nutritional habits, structure, lifestyle, and spinal hygiene. No one thing will be the magical "silver bullet" for fibromyalgia but a more comprehensive approach focused on the whole patient may result in a better outcome.

Fibromyalgia and Your Care: How's That Working for You

Dr. Phil often talks to viewers about their concerns this way. I think something can be learned from this approach when it comes to our bodily health. Perhaps you've been through the health care maze known as "fibrocare."

Many patients start off with one little problem, such as fatigue or a headache, which just seems to grow and grow, much like the entourage of doctors we collect to get answers. How many physicians did you see before being properly diagnosed? Unfortunately, most fibro sufferers endure years of misdiagnoses, years of visits to various specialists, and of course constant and widespread pain. So is it working well? Are you getting healthy? Getting back to your old healthy self? Is so, then great. If not, then read on.

Were alternatives and perhaps more natural/non-drug approaches brought to your attention? Unfortunately, the maze can be quite daunting…hard to really get a sense of any direction or what lies around the next corner.

Chiropractic care is one such alternative that remains a practical secret for many. You've seen signs for chiropractic doctors, but what do they do?

How would they approach the fibromyalgia problem? As with any health issue, it's impossible to tell what is going on and what is the best remedy without a thorough examination. I cannot speculate on your personal health. Everyone is an individual and deserves very specific attention.

What I do know is that chiropractic care does seem to improve many types of aches and pain, including those associated with fibromyalgia. Spinal pain is one of the most common symptoms.

Although I have few doubts about the importance of regular chiropractic in my own and my family's life, most patients rarely see how they could potentially benefit from such care.

Since I cannot afford to run television advertisements at prime time each night (in contrast to big drug companies), to start to change the public's perception, I send these Health Updates.

My hope is that you will be interested enough to call and discuss how my chiropractic care could be a potential solution to your fibromyalgia pains. No promises other than I will do my level best to try and help.

Fibromyalgia: What Is It And How Do Different Doctors Deal With It?

At least 2% of the United States population, or six million people, mostly women, have a diagnosis of fibromyalgia. This is a chronic (long-term) disease, which is characterized by widespread pain of at least three months duration, and includes the legs or arms and the spine. There have to be at least 11 tender spots at 18 predetermined sites on the body.

For many years, some doctors thought it was all in a patient's head and referred their patients to psychologists. Although the cause is still unknown, there is much research that shows the pains are real and quality of life is dramatically affected. In addition to the widespread pain, there are often sleep disturbances, fatigue, headaches, morning stiffness, paresthesias (tingly creepy sensations) and anxiety. All ages are affected, but most patients are middle-aged. Few have found good solutions to the problem and find themselves in a health care maze of treatments.

Although there are no guidelines for treatment, there is evidence that a multidimensional approach can help. As far as medical doctors' approach to this difficult problem, they generally use patient education and pharmacologic (medication) therapy. Although 90% of patients will take the medication approach, some have concerns about long-term use and potential undesired side effects. In the case of anti-inflammatory drugs, potential complications such as stomach bleeding can occur in some patients.

Most fibromyalgia patients use a combination of medical and alternative care because medication alone is seldom effective. Doctors of chiropractic avoid the use of medications and emphasize spinal adjustments to correct abnormal postural and motion problems. These adjustments are usually one important aspect of care often lacking for many patients. The doctor may also advise you on diet and weight-loss strategies. A low inflammation diet with lots of fruit and vegetables can help many patients. Supplements such as antioxidants and minerals are also used.

Everyone, including fibromyalgia patients, will benefit from a structured exercise program, which has both aerobic and strength-resistance training components. Although muscle pains are prominent in this disorder, lack of exercise will generally make the problem more chronic and disabling.

Fibromyalgia is a Global Problem

What do I mean by global? Well, it does occur in countries around the world, but more to the point, fibromyalgia is only one piece of a complex full-body puzzle. Patients with fibromyalgia will report widespread pain in the neck, back and in other areas, but there's also much more to the story.

Usually, patients will have sympathetic activation-stressed nerves, which can result in a depressed immune system, obesity, TMJ problems, and even high blood pressure. Headaches are also quite common, as are other aches and pains. Fibromyalgia sufferers usually have a long list of symptoms they have had over the years.

And after years of pain, most patients have avoided certain movements and exercises, thus further diminishing their quality of life.

This can all seem daunting to many doctors who want to find a pill for every pain. You may have also been prescribed antidepressants thinking this would get at this global bodily disorder.

There is not one thing that seems to help these types of patients- no silver bullet. If there were such a cure, I'd do it tomorrow.

Rather, you need to address the problem globally by correcting misalignments of the full spine and extremities, and making sure your joints are moving properly. Diet is also an issue. For many patients they will need to lose weight, and I can assist in doing this in a controlled way. Most patients need guidance about certain foods and fats that promote inflammation, which is a key point in addressing symptoms.

There may also be certain chemicals that you are ingesting that are contributing to the problem, rather than helping.

Lastly, all of my patients need to start exercising. Being a couch potato is no solution for fibromyalgia. Inactivity and inflexibility just makes joint and muscle pains worse.

I start patients off with simple daily stretches to add flexibility followed by walking. Some patients can barely get out of bed, so we start with walking to the end of the block. The goal is to get up to 15-30 minutes of fast paced walking each day. Once your weight is down to a manageable level, I encourage patients to join a gym, so they can develop more strength in all of their muscles. This comprehensive approach is key to addressing fibromyalgia symptoms, as well as other important health problems that often accompany it.

See What Our Patients Have To Say...

"Dr. David Warwick took the time to learn about my injury and recommend my options. I started with a back adjustment, and it just felt a little better immediately afterwards. I woke up the next morning and felt way better. I am now convinced I will continue my treatment until I feel completely healed. Glad I went here and met with Dr. Warwick."

"I came, hesitantly, to Dr. Warwick's office due to pain, numbness, and tingling down both arms and limited range of motion in my neck and shoulders. I was not familiar with chiropractic as a medical option, but was faced with an ongoing treatment regimen of shots in my neck and limiting my activities, possibly forever. I decided I was not ready for that and needed a more logical, natural way to return to health. Needless to say, there has been great improvement not only in my neck and shoulders, but also lower back – discomfort I had just gotten used to. Dr. Warwick's willingness to really listen and understand my interest in a natural solution to regaining my health and strength has been empowering. Dr. Warwick is a medical provider, teacher, and true healer. THANK YOU!!!

"After my auto accident I experienced frequent and mysterious headaches. But not so mysterious for Dr. Warwick. He was knowledgeable, kind, and thoughtful in explaining to me my situation. Since seeing him, my headaches are gone. I feel confident in the care Dr. Warwick skillfully provides."

"Dr. David Warwick took the time to learn about my injury and recommend my options. I started with a back adjustment, and it just felt a little better immediately afterwards. I woke up the next morning and felt way better. I am now convinced I will continue my treatment until I feel completely healed. Glad I went here and met with Dr. Warwick."

"WOW! I am pain-free for the first time in two weeks! Thanks so much to Dr. David Warwick for an amazing job. I have so far to go, but now I am on the right track. I have been telling people for years that proper setup of a guitar is crucial to it playing well, just as a front alignment and tune up is to a car. It will work without it, but nowhere near its potential. All this time, my spine has been a disaster. The first visit, I knew I was on the right track. Treated like a welcomed guest, not as a number, and walking away with less pain and increased mobility. I had forgotten it was possible! Thank you so much!"

"I went into to meet with Dr. Warwick today, having been worked on by several massage therapists and Chiropractors over the years. I had a long relationship with my chiropractor and was really just trying something new and networking (I am a massage therapist) BUT Oh MY! He adjusted me today, found things I didn't realize were going on, relieved pain I wasn't really fully aware of and changed my entire day by lifting my mood and making my stress tolerable. I ended up with a smile for several hours just because I felt AMAZING! I will be singing his praises from the mountain top, As for my other chiro, well thanks for the memories but I am now a client of Dr. Warwick! If he can do that on my first visit, I can't wait to see what regular visits will do!"

"I don't do these often, so those who know me also know how much weight this carries. Highlight of my day today was probably the most no-nonsense, hassle-free, and delightful visit to the offices of my friend Dr. David Warwick to get a checkup of my lower back pain. No lectures, no suggestions of 20 "preventive" visits, just an honest diagnosis, some great pointers, a quick and effective adjustment, and out the door I went. For anyone seeking a fantastic chiropractor, please give Dr. Warwick a call; more than a Doc, the man is a breath of fresh air!"

"Dr. David is a miracle worker!! I saw him after having no idea how I injured my back and had seen another chiropractor twice..... but within two visits Dr. David had me walking, sitting, and sleeping pain free. Thank you Dr. David...you are simply the best!!"

"I have been in pain for a very long time but I went Dr. Warwick, and he was the only one that has helped me with my lower back pain. I will continue to keep on seeing him for as long as I can. Thank you, Dr. Warwick!"

"I have never felt better in years, I have suffered from neck pain for a long time. I have had numerous doctor visits and have always still had pain. I have been seeing Dr. Warwick and was pleasantly surprised of the relief I continue to have. I love, love, love the results!"

"I came in to see Dr. Warwick because I was suffering from Bell's Palsy. Almost immediately I started seeing results. I have now been going to Dr. Warwick for 2 ½ months, and I'm 100% back. I contribute that completely to the chiropractic work I have been doing. Not only that but I found out my body was lopsided, and I feel so much better. I haven't felt this good in ten years!"

"Dr. Warwick is very kind, attentive and professional. He always asks how I am feeling and if the chiropractic work he offers is helpful to me and my health. I really appreciate his professionalism, care and knowledge. I would happily refer him to all my friends!"

"Dr. Warwick is so dedicated to your health and happiness. It has been a pleasure being treated by him and others on the staff.

I have suffered from back pain for several years. I have seen multiple chiropractors, doctors, massage therapists, and acupuncturists. I even had 3 back injections! All provided no relief. I saw Dr. Warwick ONE time and I was pain free for 12 hours, which was the first time I had been pain free in years! After 3 treatments I was pain free for a week! HIGHLY RECOMMEND!!

Today was my first time ever going into a chiropractic office, I was so nervous at first, but when Dr. David M Warwick talked to me about what was going to be done I was comfortable. He was very quick and gentle and the relief of 9 years of tension, misalignment, and stress in my neck, mid, and lower back was instantly gone. I would recommend him to anyone to go to. I seriously feel so much better for the first time in a long time thanks to him!

1st time ever to see a chiropractor & Dr. Warwick has done an amazing job with adjusting my lower back! He has been very explanatory & most of all patient with me as I learn the process for what needs to be done. I really like the option of either walking in or making an appt. online too!

I have been seeing Dr. Warwick for 9 months now. I work in a physically demanding job with a lot of repetitive motion that has taken a toll on my body. Dr. Warwick has provided me with exceptional treatment and it truly is a joy to see him knowing that I have been given back my freedom of movement and my pain is now under control. I highly recommend Dr Warwick to anyone seeking excellent chiropractic care

I felt 2 inches taller. Finally someone noticed my poor posture and recognized the pain that was there!

Dr. Warwick has been a godsend. I still play competitive baseball in my late 30's, and deal with a painful back injury, but after a visit to his office, I can not only walk out under my own power, but am ready to compete at the level I've been accustomed to my whole life. So very glad that he is here.

I was so scared to see a Chiropractor, but Dr. Warwick made my first visit very comfortable, explaining everything step by step! Now that I have gone to him a few times, I really feel like the ease of scheduling online and how AMAZING I feel after every visit is well worth the small amount of money I pay to feel great!

I feel very fortunate to have found Warwick Chiropractic. I've been to several chiropractors over the years, but Dr. Warwick's technique and bedside manner are unlike any other. He addresses all of my concerns, he listens to my needs and makes sure that I'm comfortable! I entrust him with my children's Chiropractic needs as well!

Dr. Warwick is genuine and honest. He spent time really evaluating my pain and adjusting specific to what I needed, not just the normal 3 chiropractor adjustments.

I haven't been able to lift my right arm straight up for almost a decade... after just one visit, I can reach straight up!! I'm so thankful to have found Dr. Warwick and will be back again next week for a follow up. Thank you so much!

I am grateful to Dr. Warwick for the knowledge he gave me and for his care and thoroughness in administering my alignment . This was my first visit. WOW ! WONDERFUL ! RESTORATIVE !

Dr. David Warwick at Warwick Chiropractic

Your Local Lacey / Olympia WA Chiropractor
Short Term Care for Your Back & Neck Pain
Thurston County Auto Accident Pain Relief Specialist

Walk-Ins Welcome - No Appointment Needed
Simple & Convenient On-Line Scheduling

Visit my website www.DrDavidWarwick.com
Office: 8650 Martin Way East #207, Lacey WA 98516
Call 360-951-4504

Like Us on Facebook: **Warwick Chiropractic PLLC**

Watch my YouTube Videos for Great Tips and Live Treatments
on **Warwick Chiropractic – Dr David Warwick Lacey
Chiropractor**

For More Great Articles, Visit my Blog Page
www.DrDavidWarwick.com & www.DrDavidWarwickBlog.com

Grab My FREE Relief Books
Back & Neck Pain Relief
http://backandneckpainrelieflaceychiropractor.com/
*You're Not A Dummy..Washington's Health Guide For Car Accident
Victims*
http://yourenotadummywahealthguideforcaraccidentvictims.com/

You Can Also Sign Up for my Pain Relief Email Updates & Monthly
Newsletter at www.DrDavidWarwick.com

Thank you for Subscribing to my YouTube Channel, Facebook Page,
Pain Relief Updates, and Monthly Newsletter.

Thank you for taking your time to comment and enjoy.....See You
Soon!

Questions for Dr. Warwick:

Made in the USA
Lexington, KY
15 November 2019

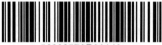